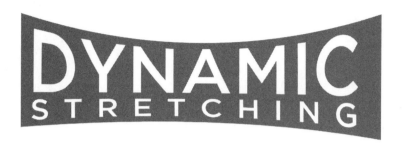

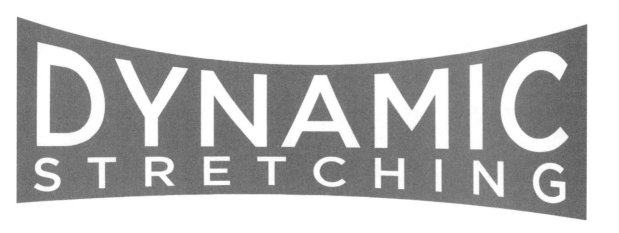

DYNAMIC STRETCHING

**THE REVOLUTIONARY NEW
WARM-UP METHOD
TO IMPROVE POWER,
PERFORMANCE AND
RANGE OF MOTION**

MARK KOVACS
Photography by **Austin Forbord**

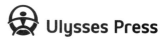
Ulysses Press

Published in the United States by Ulysses Press
P.O. Box 3440
Berkeley, CA 94703
www.ulyssespress.com

ISBN: 978-1-56975-726-0
Library of Congress Control Number 2009902021

Printed in Canada by Webcom

10 9 8 7 6 5 4

Editorial/Production	Lily Chou, Claire Chun, Abby Reser, Lauren Harrison, Judith Metzener
Index	Sayre Van Young
Interior photos	Austin Forbord/Rapt Productions
Cover design	what!design @ whatweb.com
Front cover photo	ShaneKato
Back cover photos	© istockphoto.com/mirefa (basketball), technotr (tennis), strickke (soccer)
Models	Garrett Kass, Mark Kovacs, Maria I. Martinez, Scott Mathison, Michelle Qi

Distributed by Publishers Group West

Please Note

This book has been written and published strictly for informational purposes, and in no way should be used as a substitute for consultation with health care professionals. You should not consider educational material herein to be the practice of medicine or to replace consultation with a physician or other medical practitioner. The author and publisher are providing you with information in this work so that you can have the knowledge and can choose, at your own risk, to act on that knowledge. The author and publisher also urge all readers to be aware of their health status and to consult health care professionals before beginning any health program.

table of contents

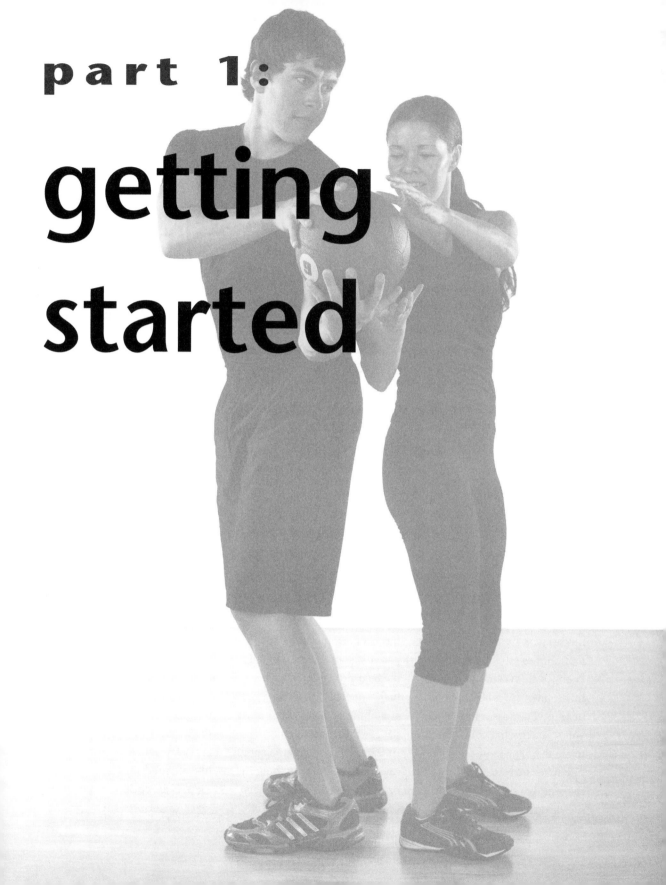

part 1:
getting
started

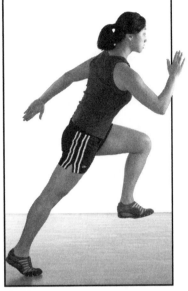

introduction

It is exercise alone that supports the spirits, and keeps the mind in vigor.

—Marcus Tullius Cicero

Sweat pours down your face. Your heart pumps out of your chest. The crowd chants an indistinct roar. Everything you've trained for your entire life comes down to less than 10 seconds. After what seems like a lifetime, the gun reverberates and the sprinters are off for the race of their lives—the 100-meter sprint in the Olympics.

You look over at the sprinter next to you and wonder if he has trained as hard as you, if his blood, sweat and tears have left stains in his T-shirts the way yours have. Stains not even bleach can fully remove.

Feet pounding on the track, the runners fly by in a blur of motion. Less than 10 seconds later, it's all over. You cross the finish line fifth while the guy next to you crosses first, and you wonder what could've made the quarter of a second difference in being on top of the world and finishing out of the medals.

One reason could've been the way you both warmed up before races: dynamic versus static stretching.

From elementary school up through the professional ranks, and even for senior athletes, the virtue of stretching has been espoused by coaches, parents, sport scientists and medical professionals. The major question is what type of stretching is best. When most people think stretching, the first image people get is someone bending and touching his or her toes, and holding this position for 15–30 seconds.

This stretch-and-hold variety is known as "static" stretching. There is great value in this traditional stretching technique, as it is relatively safe and has been shown to improve range of motion about the joint(s) being stretched. Good flexibility in all parts of the body is vital for effective sports performance, reducing the likelihood of many types of injuries and also improving the health and functionality of everyday activities. However, like all good things in life, there is an optimum time and place to perform this type of stretching, and the greatest benefits are seen when static stretching is performed *after* activity.

Over the last decade, researchers, coaches and medical professionals have found that there are more optimum methods to warm up for physical activity, and that the traditional static stretching routine before sports should be replaced with a more dynamic activity that can also provide a number of other benefits to the athletes. "Dynamic warm-ups" and "dynamic stretches" are the terms used throughout the book to describe exercises and movement patterns that are great to perform before physical activity and can help improve performance and reduce the likelihood of injury in both the short and long term.

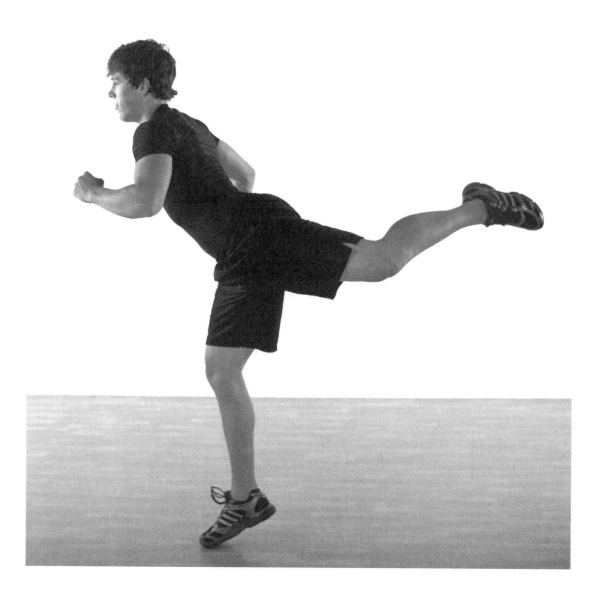

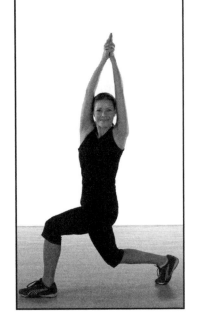

what is dynamic stretching?

Over the last decade, a lot of information and misinformation has been disseminated through the media, coaches, trainers, athletes and parents about the positives and negatives of stretching.

Much of this information is very good, practical and useful, yet stretching is still an area of training that is not that well understood compared to the other major areas of athletic performance, such as speed, endurance or strength training.

Part of the difficulty with the information that is available on stretching is the inconsistent use of terminology and the fact that many coaches and trainers use different words to describe the same types of stretching. This terminology will be explained in more detail in the next section.

The best way to think of the difference between dynamic stretching activities versus traditional static stretching activities is that in the dynamic movements, once the muscle is lengthened, a contraction occurs and the muscles, joints, tendons and ligaments have to provide force in this stretched position, creating greater functional ability in these extended ranges of motion. Some good examples are the walking lunge with rotation and the hamstring handwalk. Both of these exercises require a combination of strength and flexibility, and are a perfect way to increase strength, flexibility, balance and coordination while also warming up before a sport or specific physical activity. The use of dynamic activities during the warm-up period provides greater "bang for your buck," with more benefits than that of a static routine.

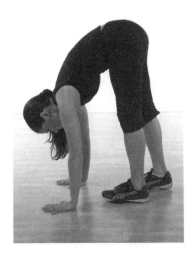

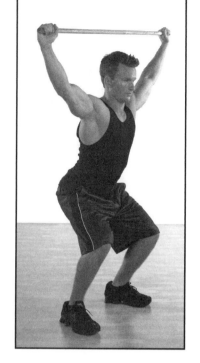

under-standing the terms

As mentioned earlier, the biggest difficulty regarding flexibility is the inconsistency with terms. Let's define some of the major terms that will be used throughout this book. This section provides an easy-to-understand reference based on the most commonly accepted principles.

Warm-Up

An effective warm-up will increase muscle temperature and the body's core temperature, and improve blood flow through the entire system. A warm-up period is important before any athletic event or performance. There should be multiple goals for the warm-up, including preparing the athlete both physically and mentally for the physical activity and/or competition ahead. Successful warm-ups should provide the following positive results as outlined in the *National Strength and Conditioning Association's Essentials of Strength Training and Conditioning*:

- Faster muscle contraction and relaxation of both agonist (contracting) and antagonist (relaxing) muscles
- Improvement in the rate of force development and reaction time
- Improvement in muscle strength and power
- Lower resistance in the muscles
- Improved oxygen delivery via an increase in temperature
- Increased blood flow to active muscles
- Enhanced metabolic reactions that result in greater fuel utilization.

Range of Motion

Range of motion is the degree of movement that occurs at a joint. For athletes, it's important to have functional or sport-specific range of motion in the plane of motion, and movement patterns that the athlete uses during practice or competition.

Flexibility

Flexibility is the measure of range of motion and has both static and dynamic components. Static flexibility is the range of movement about a joint and its surrounding muscles, ligaments and connective tissue during a passive movement. *Static flexibility* requires no voluntary muscle activity. The force produced for stretch comes from an external source such as a partner, gravity or a machine. *Dynamic flexibility* is the available range of motion during active movements and therefore requires voluntary muscle actions. An athlete's range of motion is typically greater dynamically than statically.

Stretching

There are three major types of stretching that have been performed prior to sporting activities: static, dynamic and ballistic. *Static stretching* is a constant stretch held at an end point for anywhere between 15 seconds and 5 minutes.

Dynamic stretching is an activity-specific functional stretching exercise that should utilize sport-specific (or activity-specific) movements to prepare the body for activity. Dynamic stretching focuses on movement patterns requiring a combination of muscles, joints and planes of motion, whereas static stretching typically focuses on a single muscle group, joint and plane of motion.

Ballistic stretching involves active muscle effort and uses a bouncing-type movement to increase the range without holding the stretch at an end position. Unlike static stretching, ballistic stretching triggers the stretch reflex and can increase the likelihood of injury in individuals who have not progressed appropriately or do not have the correct training background for this form of stretching. Ballistic stretching is typically not recommended as a component of an effective warm-up for the vast majority of the population. It should be avoided by individuals with a history of lower back and/or hamstring injuries.

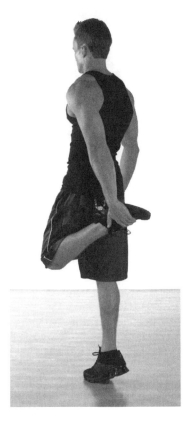

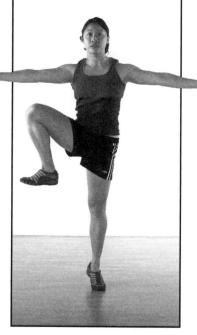

why dynamic stretching?

The warm-up should not be used purely as a time to increase body temperature before more strenuous activity. If this were the only purpose of the warm-up, then jumping rope, jogging or riding a stationary bike would be enough to prepare for athletic performance.

The warm-up is a time that can be used to gain numerous training adaptations in many aspects of physical conditioning. These benefits can include improved strength, flexibility, muscular endurance, coordination and the correction of major and minor muscle imbalances. A great aspect of an effective dynamic warm-up is that it can be a complete total-body workout for athletes with time constraints; if performed correctly, this warm-up can result in positive training adaptations to improve per-

formance. The dynamic warm-up can be a time to focus on improving strength, power, speed and agility.

Recreational athletes typically perform a dynamic warm-up of 10 to 20 minutes, but the more advanced an athlete becomes, the more time should be spent on the warm-up. It's not uncommon for professional athletes to spend 30 to 60 minutes focused on the warm-up. The warm-up provides multiple benefits to the athlete in addition to warming the body for future

activity; it's a specific workout in itself and many of the activities mimic movements and muscle recruitment patterns of the sport.

The Myths Surrounding Pre-Exercise Static Stretching

Pre-exercise static stretching has been used by coaches and athletes for decades in the hope of improving performance and preventing injuries. In the 1980s and mid-'90s, it had been suggested in scientific literature as a good addition to athletes' warm-up before physical activity.[1, 2] Since the early 1990s, many researchers from Japan to Australia to the U.S. have been performing studies on stretching, looking at the best methods to improve athletic performance. This section summarizes some of the research on stretching, performance and injury prevention, but if the science behind stretching is of interest to you, a detailed reference section is included at the end of the book to guide you to some of the most beneficial studies in this area.

Despite early evidence in the 1960s that static stretching prior to activity did not improve sprinting performance,[3] static stretching has been a common practice by most coaches and athletes in warm-up routines for physical activity. However, contrary to the typical belief that static stretching improves physical performance, there have been numerous studies that demonstrate that traditional static stretching actually has the reverse effect. It can decrease performance in strength, speed and power activities.[3-14] Depth-jump performance (when an athletes jumps from a small height to the ground and then explosively jumps up again),

which is a good practical indication of power output, is significantly reduced following static stretching.[11, 13] Vertical jump height has also been significantly reduced when prior static stretching was used.[12, 14] Research studies on strength and power performances following static stretching have shown decreases in immediate performance by as much as 30 percent.[4, 5, 7-9] This can have a tremendous influence on performance, especially in sports that require quick, explosive bursts of power and strength, such as sprints, jumps and throws in track and field, short distance swimming events, Olympic weightlifting, powerlifting and bodybuilding.

The deficit in performance following static stretching may be dependent on the type of stretching and mode of activity that follows the stretching routine. The deficit in performance following static stretching has been shown to last approximately 60 minutes after the stretching routine.[9] Researchers around the world are studying the exact cause of this decrease in performance. There are theories as to why it reduces performance but, as of this writing, no definitive mechanism has been verified. Some of the theories include changes in reflex sensitivity, muscle/

BENEFITS OF A DYNAMIC WARM-UP

- Stretching
- Power
- Endurance
- Flexibility
- Coordination
- Balance
- Neuromuscular activation
- Speed
- Mental preparation

tendon stiffness and/or neuromuscular activation.[9, 13, 15, 16]

The positive or negative effect on performance after static stretching may be dependent on the speed of movement of the exercise involved. Reduced performance has not been shown when high-velocity movements were undertaken after a static stretching routine.[17] For instance, the static stretching routine had no effect on either speed or accuracy (performance) of an explosive tennis serve.[17] A suggested reason for why static stretching prior to the tennis serve did not reduce performance, as had been seen in other studies, was that the pre-activity stretching may not decrease performance in high-speed and/or accuracy-related movements.[17] The authors refer to a study that showed results of significant reductions in isokinetic strength, but only at low speeds of joint rotation.[5] However, this theory has not always been supported, as was seen in a recent study on sprint speed times (which involves high-speed explosive movements) over 20 meters in highly trained athletes. It was found that, compared to no stretching, static stretching significantly reduced performance by increasing sprint speed times.[10]

It appears clear from the numerous studies performed that pre-activity static stretching reduces physical performance in strength, speed and power activities.[3, 4, 7-16] Therefore, athletes that perform sports that require strength, speed or power should limit or avoid slow static stretching within about an hour of training or competition. These academic studies, along with the years of coaching practice that have found a limitation on performance with static stretching, provide another reason why performing dynamic warm-ups offer a great benefit for improved athletic performance. This improvement in performance is highlighted in sports that rely heavily on strength, speed or power.

Apart from the traditional and sometimes misinformed belief that pre-exercise static stretching improves perform-

ance, a second major reason that many coaches and athletes still perform static stretching before activity is the notion that it may help in reducing the likelihood of injury. This may be based on the notion that a "tight" muscle-tendon unit is less compliant, which means that it cannot be stretched to as great a degree.[18, 19] This assumption has resulted in the long-held belief that stretching may prevent muscle- and tendon-related injuries.[18] However, the current research does not provide substantial support for this assumption and there is information that supports the opposing view that pre-activity static stretching may not reduce the risk of injury.[18-29]

A study looking at the prevention of lower-limb injuries in 1,538 male army recruits found that pre-exercise static stretching had no effect on injury rates after a 12-week stretching protocol.[20] A 2001 review of stretching studies found that there was no clear evidence to support the notion that pre-activity stretching exercises were effective in preventing lower limb injuries.[29] The large majority of studies and review articles on stretching and injury rates have found no link between pre-activity

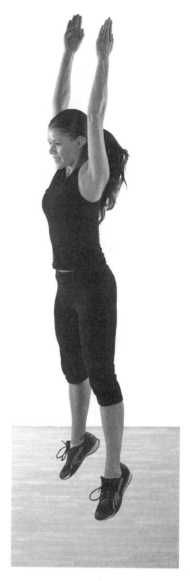

static stretching and a reduction in injury rates.[18, 19, 22, 24-30]

It must be mentioned that static stretching, although not showing a relationship with a reduction in injury rates, has not been shown to increase the risk of injuries either. The cause of injuries in sport and physical activity is multifaceted, and flexibility is only one area that may improve/reduce

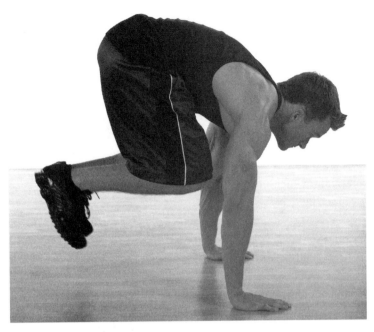

the likelihood of injury. Fatigue[31] and volume of exercise[32] have both been suggested as a predisposing factor to physically induced muscle injury. It's important to warm up appropriately and train effectively and efficiently while recovering optimally to aid in the prevention of injuries. Dynamic warm-ups increase core temperature to a greater extent than static stretching–focused warm-ups. This provides an improved protective mechanism against muscle strains and joint sprains, which are more prevalent when the body is cool. Dynamic warm-ups that mimic the movement patterns and speed of movement that the sport will impose on the body

also help to reduce the likelihood of injury as the movement patterns and ranges of motion encountered during the sport have been trained during the warm-up. This mimicking of the sporting movements is not accomplished with static stretching.

Practical Application for Athletes at All Levels

From the available research, it appears that static stretching within an hour of practice or competition does not improve performance and was not shown to reduce the risk of injury. However, limited or poor muscle and joint range of motion *can* reduce performance and increase the risk of injury.[33] Therefore, it's impera-

tive that athletes at all levels and ages improve range of motion and flexibility in the major muscles and joints of the body. A good time for athletes to perform static stretching exercises is post-exercise[34, 35] and/or in the evenings. Performing stretching activities at the end of workouts provides similar improvements in range of motion as performing them at other times.[36] The dynamic warm-up activities that are outlined in this book have been shown by research to be more beneficial and specific, as well as produce greater results, in improving physical performance.[1, 35, 37-40]

Now that we have a better understanding about what the science tells us about traditional static stretching, it's time to learn the greatest warm-up and dynamic stretching exercises available to improve athletic performance, health and overall well-being.

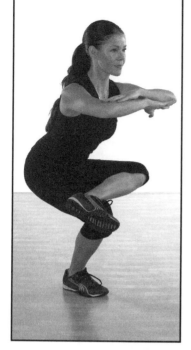

before you begin

This book is intended to be a comprehensive guide to dynamic warm-up exercises and routines for a wide variety of sports. Before you begin undertaking any type of physical activity, including dynamic warm-up exercises, it's important that you have medical clearance from a physician and that you follow the principle of progressive overload.

Progressive overload is the concept of systematically and gradually increasing the intensity and volume of the warm-up routines. The intensity of the warm-up activity includes the range of motion, force and velocity of movement. The *volume* includes the number of repetitions and/or the total time.

Beginner athletes who have little training or competition experience should start with movements that involve smaller ranges of motion, lower force requirements and slower velocities of movement. The walking lunge is an example of a beginner exercise, whereas the bent-leg bound is an advanced exercise with a greater range of motion, higher force and faster velocity of movement. Ten yards is a good starting distance for most of these movements, but more advanced athletes many times perform these movement patterns over distances of 20 to 40 yards.

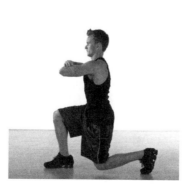

Walking lunge

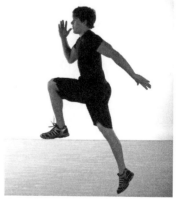

Bent-leg bound

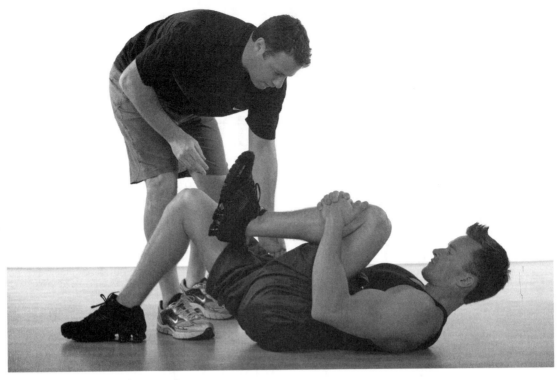

Author Mark Kovacs makes an adjustment.

Before beginning the warm-up, you should perform a light aerobic activity for 3 to 10 minutes to slowly increase your heart rate and muscle and body temperature. Simple exercises like jogging, riding a stationary bike or jump roping are all good, quick ways to prepare your body for the next stage of the session. It's recommended that intensity or total volume is not increased by more than 5 to 10 percent per week. This will help prevent the possibility of progressing too aggressively and increasing the potential for injury.

The sample programs for different sports outlined in this book (pages 21–46) provide a good starting point to help you progress your dynamic warm-ups. These programs are structured in a way that progresses from less challenging to more challenging exercises. As you develop your strength, flexibility, power, balance, coordination, speed and endurance, you can develop your own warm-up routines from the 50-plus exercises provided throughout the book.

Playing It Safe

Too many athletes, especially young ones, go through the motions of various exercises and don't focus on correct technique. Without a focus on technique, many of the benefits of a structured dynamic warm-up are not achieved. This book provides both written instructions and photographs for each exercise and movement pattern, making it a useful tool in learning and continually refining the technique of each exercise. Since it's important to concentrate on "feeling" the muscles that are the focus of each exercise and consciously attempt to recruit those muscles, each exercise in this book lists the major muscles that should be recruited during the exercise. Technique is very important in these movements as it will help develop the correct muscles and movement patterns; in addition, it will also limit the likelihood of injury. So take up the challenge and make your dynamic warm-up routines an integral part of your exercise or sport session.

Train smart, work hard and achieve athletic success.

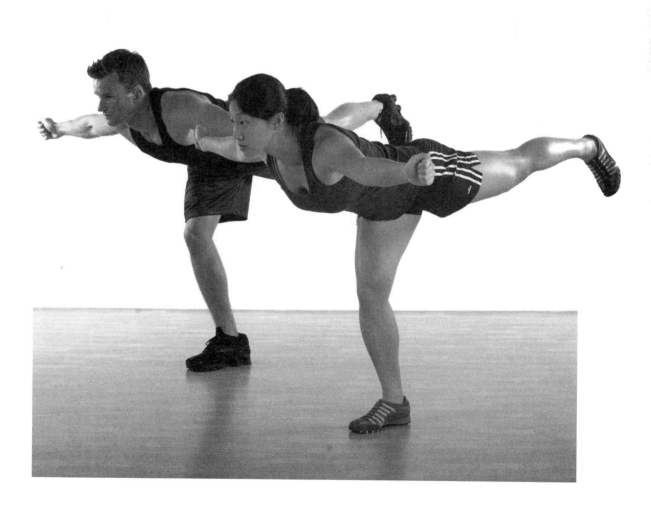

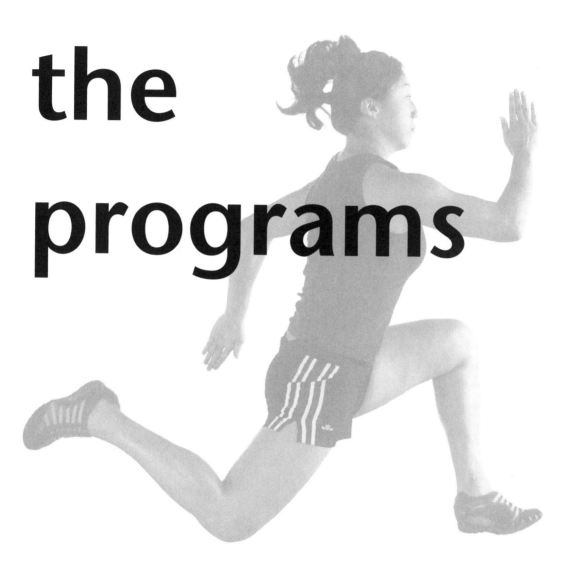

part 2:
the
programs

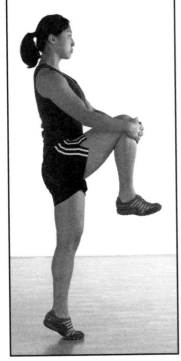

how to use this book

This book features dozens of different exercises and warm-up routines for different muscles, movements and sports. These exercises can also be combined in individualized programs based on your specific needs. Use these exercises as warm-ups, active recovery exercises, or even total-body workouts.

The uses of these movements are numerous. For most athletes, performing 10–15 exercises during a 15-minute warm-up before sports practice or competition is the most common method of applying these exercises to improve performance. Many elite and professional athletes commonly perform these exercises for 45 minutes before training or competition. For individuals coming back from injuries, or to improve functional strength and flexibility, it's not uncommon for these exercises to be performed as the entire training session.

The great thing about these exercises is that most require no equipment and very little space, and can be progressed consistently as you become stronger, more flexible and able to maintain greater muscular endurance. Performing a dynamic stretching session most, if not all, days of the week will aid in improving athletic performance, reducing the likelihood of injury and also providing added benefits to tasks of daily living. Remember that all exercises should be performed using a strict focus on technique and excellent body posture in the upper, lower and core regions of the body. The exercise descriptions in Part 3 of the book provide short, easy-to-understand descriptions to help you focus on performing each movement with the perfect technique to achieve the stated objective.

BASEBALL/SOFTBALL

Baseball and softball are sports that require high levels of rotational strength and flexibility. Hitting a baseball/softball requires an effective kinetic chain transfer from the ground up through the lower body, through the core and out through the arms into the bat, which allows for powerful ball contact. Warm-ups should focus on rotational movements for hitting, but also linear movements for base running.

Recreational Athletes: Perform one set per session.   *Elite Athletes:* Perform two sets per session.

	PAGE	EXERCISE	DISTANCE/REPS
	p. 49	Heel Walk	10 yards
	p. 51	Knee to Chest Walk	10 yards
	p. 57	Hamstring Handwalk—Inchworm	10 yards
	p. 58	Spiderman Crawl	10 yards
	p. 62	Rotational Walking Lunge	20 yards
	p. 68	Sumo Squat Walk	10 yards
	p. 98	Carioca	20 yards
	p. 84	A-Walk, Skip, Run Progression	20 yards
	p. 102	Hugs	10 yards
	p. 103	Cheerleaders	10 yards
	p. 104	Wipers	10 yards
	p. 94	Burpee Sprint	10 yards

BASKETBALL

Basketball places a major emphasis on acceleration, change of direction, and jumping ability. Therefore, warm-ups need to focus on these areas, with a gradual progression from less intense movements to highly explosive movements in multiple planes of motion (forward, backward, side-to-side and vertical).

Recreational Athletes: Perform one set per session.   *Elite Athletes:* Perform two sets per session.

	PAGE	EXERCISE	DISTANCE/REPS
	p. 48	Toe Walk	10 yards
	p. 49	Heel Walk	10 yards
	p. 50	Side Ankle Walk	10 yards
	p. 85	Overhead Squat	10 reps
	p. 57	Hamstring Handwalk—Inchworm	20 yards
	p. 58	Spiderman Crawl	10 yards
	p. 84	A-Walk, Skip, Run Progression	20 reps
	p. 75	Split Jumps/Lunge Jumps	20 reps
	p. 81	Jump Jump Sprint	10 yards
	p. 82	Backpedal	10 yards
	p. 96	10-Yard Movement Sequence	10 yards
	p. 104	Wipers	10 yards

BODYBUILDING

Bodybuilding emphasizes size, thickness, symmetry and low body fat. The warm-up exercises for bodybuilding need to focus on all the muscles of the body; the goal is to reduce the likelihood of injury. These exercises can be performed as "cardio" as well.

Recreational Athletes: Perform one set per session.　　　*Elite Athletes: Perform two sets per session.*

	PAGE	EXERCISE	DISTANCE/REPS
	p. 48	Toe Walk	10 yards
	p. 85	Overhead Squat	10 reps
	p. 52	Walking Quad Stretch	10 yards
	p. 71	Glute Ham Bridge	10 yards
	p. 54	One-Leg Walking Opposite—Ostrich	20 yards
	p. 65	Knee-to-Chest Hold into Lunge	10 yards
	p. 66	Lateral Lunge	20 reps
	p. 70	Figure-4 Squat	20 reps
	p. 69	Low Squat Walk	10 yards
	p. 78	Concentric Squat Jumps	10 yards
	p. 102	Hugs	10 yards
	p. 104	Wipers	10 yards

CYCLING

Cycling is a lower body–focused activity that requires strength in the quadriceps, hamstrings and calf muscles. The core needs to be strong to help with transition of force through the lower body into the pedals. Hip flexor and hamstring flexibility is vital for efficient pedal cadence and efficiency of movement throughout each pedal cycle.

Recreational Athletes: Perform one set per session.   *Elite Athletes: Perform two sets per session.*

	PAGE	EXERCISE	DISTANCE/REPS
	p. 48	Toe Walk	10 yards
	p. 49	Heel Walk	10 yards
	p. 67	Overhead Squat Progression	10 reps
	p. 57	Hamstring Handwalk—Inchworm	10 yards
	p. 58	Spiderman Crawl	10 yards
	p. 105	Scorpion	10 yards
	p. 52	Walking Quad Stretch	10 yards
	p. 65	Knee-to-Chest Hold into Lunge	20 yards
	p. 70	Figure-4 Squat	10 yards
	p. 78	Concentric Squat Jumps	5 reps
	p. 77	Repeated Squat Jumps	5 reps
	p. 87	Bent-Leg Bound	20 yards

FIELD HOCKEY

Field hockey requires similar movements to soccer. Acceleration, change of direction and deceleration ability are paramount for success on the field. Linear and lateral movements are needed, and hamstring flexibility is very important to reduce the likelihood of hamstring and lower back injuries.

Recreational Athletes: Perform one set per session.   *Elite Athletes:* Perform two sets per session.

	PAGE	EXERCISE	DISTANCE/REPS
	p. 48	Toe Walk	10 yards
	p. 49	Heel Walk	10 yards
	p. 50	Side Ankle Walk	10 yards
	p. 57	Hamstring Handwalk—Inchworm	10 yards
	p. 58	Spiderman Crawl	10 yards
	p. 59	Straight-Leg March	10 yards
	p. 66	Lateral Lunge*	10 yards
	p. 62	Rotational Walking Lunge	10 yards
	p. 69	Low Squat Walk	10 yards
	p. 84	A-Walk, Skip, Run Progression	20 yards
	p. 86	B-Walk, Skip, Run Progression	20 yards
	p. 93	Triple Jump Sprint	20 yards

*Add Hugs, Wipers and/or Cheerleaders to lunge exercise to warm-up upper body as well.

FOOTBALL, AUSTRALIAN RULES

In Australian rules football, large distances must be covered in short amounts of time. Maximal-velocity sprinting is common. Therefore, it's important to improve hamstring and lower back range of motion as well as core strength for fast, explosive change-of-direction movements.

Recreational Athletes: Perform one set per session.　　*Elite Athletes:* Perform two sets per session.

	PAGE	EXERCISE	DISTANCE/REPS
	p. 48	Toe Walk	10 yards
	p. 49	Heel Walk	10 yards
	p. 50	Side Ankle Walk	10 yards
	p. 52	Walking Quad Stretch	10 yards
	p. 57	Hamstring Handwalk—Inchworm	10 yards
	p. 59	Straight-Leg March	10 yards
	p. 58	Spiderman Crawl	10 yards
	p. 60	Linear Walking Lunge	20 yards
	p. 66	Lateral Lunge	10 yards
	p. 80	High-Knee Run	20 yards
	p. 86	B-Walk, Skip, Run Progression	20 yards
	p. 93	Triple Jump Sprint	20 yards

FOOTBALL—SKILL POSITIONS

Skill positions such as running backs, wide receivers and corner backs require explosive acceleration with rapid change of direction and deceleration abilities. As hip flexor and hamstring range of motion are vital to improve speed and reduce the likelihood of the most common injuries to skill position players, these muscles need to be a focus of the warm-up period.

Recreational Athletes: Perform one set per session.   *Elite Athletes:* Perform two sets per session.

	PAGE	EXERCISE	DISTANCE/REPS
	p. 48	Toe Walk	10 yards
	p. 49	Heel Walk	10 yards
	p. 50	Side Ankle Walk	10 yards
	p. 57	Hamstring Handwalk—Inchworm	10 yards
	p. 58	Spiderman Crawl	10 yards
	p. 66	Lateral Lunge	20 yards
	p. 79	Power Skips	10 yards
	p. 84	A-Walk, Skip, Run Progression	10 yards
	p. 92	Squat Jump Sprint	10 yards
	p. 96	10-Yard Movement Sequence	20 yards
	p. 88	Straight-Leg Bound	20 yards
	pp. 102–104	Hugs/Cheerleaders/Wipers Combo	10 yards

FOOTBALL—LINEMAN

The line positions in football require explosive power predominantly in a linear direction, but there is also a need for quick lateral movements. Upper body strength and flexibility, especially in the wrists and forearm, are a focus, as well as hip flexor range of motion to help with acceleration and lower body power production.

Recreational Athletes: *Perform one set per session.*   **Elite Athletes:** *Perform two sets per session.*

	PAGE	EXERCISE	DISTANCE/REPS
	p. 49	Heel Walk	10 yards
	p. 50	Side Ankle Walk	10 yards
	p. 57	Hamstring Handwalk—Inchworm	10 yards
	p. 58	Spiderman Crawl	10 yards
	p. 53	Knee to Shoulder Lateral Walk—Frogger	10 yards
	p. 69	Low Squat Walk	10 yards
	p. 66	Lateral Lunge	10 yards
	p. 70	Figure-4 Squat	10 yards
	p. 56	Upper Body Handwalk	10 yards
	p. 68	Sumo Squat Walk	10 yards
	p. 96	10-Yard Movement Sequence	10 yards
	pp. 102–104	Hugs/Cheerleaders/Wipers Combo	10 yards

GOLF

Golf requires very large rotational forces and single-effort power movements. Dynamic range of motion at the trunk, hips, core and shoulder girdle are vital to improved performance and reduction in injury. Warm-ups for golf need to focus heavily on rotation in both the upper and lower body, as well as core stabilization during all movements.

Recreational Athletes: *Perform one set per session.*   **Elite Athletes:** *Perform two sets per session.*

	PAGE	EXERCISE	DISTANCE/REPS
	p. 50	Side Ankle Walk	10 yards
	p. 71	Glute Ham Bridge	10 yards
	p. 67	Overhead Squat Progression	10 yards
	p. 57	Hamstring Handwalk—Inchworm	10 yards
	p. 58	Spiderman Crawl	10 yards
	p. 62	Rotational Walking Lunge	10 yards
	pp. 102–104	Hugs/Cheerleaders/Wipers Combo	10 yards
	p. 101	Dynamic Empty Can	10 yards
	p. 78	Concentric Squat Jumps	10 yards
	p. 56	Upper Body Handwalk	10 yards
	p. 72	Lateral Pass	10 yards
	p. 76	Countermovement Squat Jumps	10 yards

GYMNASTICS

Gymnastics is a sport that has many different components (e.g., horse, pommel horse, vault, uneven bars, rings, floor routines, etc.). The athlete's overall range of motion is highly valued, and explosiveness in multiple directions needs to be a focus of warm-ups.

Recreational Athletes: *Perform one set per session.*　　　　**Elite Athletes:** *Perform two sets per session.*

	PAGE	EXERCISE	DISTANCE/REPS
	p. 49	Heel Walk	10 yards
	p. 51	Knee to Chest Walk	10 yards
	p. 57	Hamstring Handwalk—Inchworm	10 yards
	p. 58	Spiderman Crawl	10 yards
	p. 62	Rotational Walking Lunge	10 yards
	p. 68	Sumo Squat Walk	10 yards
	p. 98	Carioca	20 yards
	p. 101	Dynamic Empty Can	10 yards
	p. 102	Hugs	10 yards
	p. 103	Cheerleaders	10 yards
	p. 104	Wipers	10 yards
	p. 73	Overhead Pass	10 yards

ICE HOCKEY

Hockey (both on ice and on in-line skates) places a large emphasis on the core and lower body strength, power and range of motion. The ability to change direction quickly and produce explosive lateral movements are also paramount to success. Hockey warm-ups need to focus on lateral movements and the improvement of rotational range of motion to prepare hockey players for high-level performance.

Recreational Athletes: Perform one set per session.   *Elite Athletes: Perform two sets per session.*

	PAGE	EXERCISE	DISTANCE/REPS
	p. 49	Heel Walk	10 yards
	p. 57	Hamstring Handwalk—Inchworm	10 yards
	p. 58	Spiderman Crawl	10 yards
	p. 105	Scorpion	10 yards
	p. 66	Lateral Lunge	10 yards
	p. 70	Figure-4 Squat	20 yards
	p. 66	Lateral Lunge	10 yards
	p. 72	Lateral Pass	10 yards
	p. 100	High-Knee Lateral Skip	10 yards
	p. 96	10-Yard Movement Sequence	10 yards
	p. 87	Bent-Leg Bound	20 yards
	pp. 102–104	Hugs/Cheerleaders/Wipers Combo	10 yards

LACROSSE

Lacrosse athletes require a combination of upper body, lower body and core strength in all planes of motion due to the simultaneous use of upper and lower body for running, catching and throwing. The warm-up routine for lacrosse needs to focus on these multi-joint and multi-plane movements.

Recreational Athletes: *Perform one set per session.*   ***Elite Athletes:*** *Perform two sets per session.*

	PAGE	EXERCISE	DISTANCE/REPS
	p. 48	Toe Walk	10 yards
	p. 49	Heel Walk	10 yards
	p. 50	Side Ankle Walk	10 yards
	p. 57	Hamstring Handwalk—Inchworm	10 yards
	p. 58	Spiderman Crawl	10 yards
	p. 61	Straight-Leg Walking Lunge	10 yards
	p. 66	Lateral Lunge*	10 yards
	p. 62	Rotational Walking Lunge	10 yards
	p. 84	A-Walk, Skip, Run Progression	10 yards
	p. 56	Upper Body Handwalk	10 yards
	p. 93	Triple Jump Sprint	20 yards

*Add Hugs, Wipers and/or Cheerleaders to lunge exercise to warm-up upper body as well.

RACQUETBALL/SQUASH

Both squash and racquetball have similar physical requirements and need explosive lower body movements in multiple directions. They also require kinetic chain energy transfer through the ground up and into the strokes. The utilization of rotational strength and range of motion is paramount to success and these components need to be incorporated during the warm-up period.

Recreational Athletes: Perform one set per session.   *Elite Athletes: Perform two sets per session.*

	PAGE	EXERCISE	DISTANCE/REPS
	p. 49	Heel Walk	10 yards
	p. 50	Side Ankle Walk	10 yards
	p. 85	Overhead Squat	10 yards
	p. 57	Hamstring Handwalk—Inchworm	10 yards
	p. 58	Spiderman Crawl	10 yards
	p. 69	Low Squat Walk	10 yards
	p. 84	A-Walk, Skip, Run Progression	10 yards
	p. 56	Upper Body Handwalk	10 yards
	p. 62	Rotational Walking Lunge*	10 yards
	p. 77	Repeated Squat Jumps	10 yards
	p. 96	10-Yard Movement Sequence	10 yards
	p. 90	Quick Feet Sprint	10 yards

*Add Hugs, Wipers and/or Cheerleaders to lunge exercise to warm-up upper body as well.

RUGBY

Rugby is a sport that requires a combination of power, strength, agility, speed and endurance. Therefore, warm-ups for rugby require movements in all planes of motion. Lateral, linear and multi-directional activities should be incorporated, and multiple distances need to be trained, from acceleration to maximum velocity movements.

Recreational Athletes: Perform one set per session.   *Elite Athletes: Perform two sets per session.*

	PAGE	EXERCISE	DISTANCE/REPS
	p. 48	Toe Walk	10 yards
	p. 49	Heel Walk	10 yards
	p. 50	Side Ankle Walk	10 yards
	p. 57	Hamstring Handwalk—Inchworm	10 yards
	p. 58	Spiderman Crawl	10 yards
	p. 105	Scorpion	10 yards
	p. 66	Lateral Lunge	10 yards
	p. 64	Elbow to Knee Lunge	10 yards
	p. 69	Low Squat Walk	10 yards
	p. 84	A-Walk, Skip, Run Progression	20 yards
	p. 86	B-Walk, Skip, Run Progression	20 yards
	p. 93	Triple Jump Sprint	20 yards

SKIING

Alpine and Nordic skiing both emphasize linear acceleration with some lateral movement. Warm-ups for skiing should focus on flexibility as well as power in linear and lateral planes for improved overall physical performance.

Recreational Athletes: Perform one set per session.   *Elite Athletes: Perform two sets per session.*

	PAGE	EXERCISE	DISTANCE/REPS
	p. 48	Toe Walk	10 yards
	p. 49	Heel Walk	10 yards
	p. 50	Side Ankle Walk	10 yards
	p. 57	Hamstring Handwalk—Inchworm	10 yards
	p. 58	Spiderman Crawl	10 yards
	p. 66	Lateral Lunge	10 yards
	p. 79	Power Skips	20 yards
	p. 77	Repeated Squat Jumps	10 yards
	p. 92	Squat Jump Sprint	10 yards
	p. 96	10-Yard Movement Sequence	10 yards
	p. 87	Bent-Leg Bound	20 yards
	p. 101	Dynamic Empty Can	10 yards

SOCCER

Soccer is a sport that requires a focus on multi-directional movement through all planes of motion. The warm-ups need to focus on dynamic range-of-motion exercises to help prevent injuries, especially in the lower back, hips, hamstrings and hip flexors.

Recreational Athletes: Perform one set per session.   *Elite Athletes: Perform two sets per session.*

PAGE	EXERCISE	DISTANCE/REPS
p. 49	Heel Walk	10 yards
p. 50	Side Ankle Walk	10 yards
p. 52	Walking Quad Stretch	10 yards
p. 57	Hamstring Handwalk—Inchworm	10 yards
p. 58	Spiderman Crawl	10 yards
p. 60	Linear Walking Lunge	10 yards
p. 66	Lateral Lunge	10 yards
p. 79	Power Skips	20 yards
p. 84	A-Walk, Skip, Run Progression	20 yards
p. 86	B-Walk, Skip, Run Progression	20 yards
p. 98	Carioca	20 yards
p. 93	Triple Jump Sprint	20 yards

SWIMMING

Swimming, both long and short distances, requires a combination of upper and lower body power with great core strength to help with effective energy transfer through the water. The warm-up period for swimming can be performed both on land and in the water.

Recreational Athletes: Perform one set per session.   *Elite Athletes: Perform two sets per session.*

	PAGE	EXERCISE	DISTANCE/REPS
	p. 48	Toe Walk	10 yards
	p. 49	Heel Walk	10 yards
	p. 85	Overhead Squat	10 yards
	p. 57	Hamstring Handwalk—Inchworm	10 yards
	p. 58	Spiderman Crawl	10 yards
	p. 53	Knee to Shoulder Lateral Walk—Frogger	10 yards
	p. 66	Lateral Lunge	10 yards
	p. 56	Upper Body Handwalk	10 yards
	p. 101	Dynamic Empty Can	10 yards
	p. 96	10-Yard Movement Sequence	10 yards
	pp. 102–104	Hugs/Cheerleaders/Wipers Combo	10 yards
	p. 73	Overhead Pass	10 yards

TENNIS

Tennis requires a combination of flexibility, power, strength and dynamic balance to perform at a high level. The energy transfer from the ground up through the kinetic chain requires a strong core and effective strength and flexibility through the lower body, up through the core and upper body and into the racquet. Dynamic range of motion at the hips (both linear and lateral) and shoulder area is vital to help prevent the likelihood of injury.

Recreational Athletes: Perform one set per session.   *Elite Athletes: Perform two sets per session.*

	PAGE	EXERCISE	DISTANCE/REPS
	p. 49	Heel Walk	10 yards
	p. 57	Hamstring Handwalk—Inchworm	10 yards
	p. 74	Ankle Flips	10 yards
	p. 58	Spiderman Crawl	10 yards
	p. 53	Knee to Shoulder Lateral Walk—Frogger	10 yards
	p. 66	Lateral Lunge	10 yards
	p. 95	Lateral Shuffle	10 yards
	p. 102	Rotational Walking Lunge	10 yards
	p. 72	Lateral Pass	10 yards
	p. 96	10-Yard Movement Sequence	10 yards
	p. 101	Dynamic Empty Can	10 yards
	pp. 102–104	Hugs/Cheerleaders/Wipers Combo	10 yards

TRACK AND FIELD—DISTANCE

Distance events require a warm-up that focuses on linear movements with appropriate flexibility in the lower body and appropriate core strength to aid in efficiency of movement, which will result in less energy used per stride.

Recreational Athletes: Perform one set per session.   *Elite Athletes: Perform two sets per session.*

	PAGE	EXERCISE	DISTANCE/REPS
	p. 48	Toe Walk	10 yards
	p. 49	Heel Walk	10 yards
	p. 50	Side Ankle Walk	10 yards
	p. 89	Ankle Taps	10 yards
	p. 57	Hamstring Handwalk—Inchworm	10 yards
	p. 58	Spiderman Crawl	10 yards
	p. 105	Scorpion	10 yards
	p. 79	Power Skips	20 yards
	p. 77	Repeated Squat Jumps	10 yards
	p. 83	Backward Run	10 yards
	p. 84	A-Walk, Skip, Run Progression	20 yards
	p. 86	B-Walk, Skip, Run Progression	40 yards

TRACK AND FIELD—SPRINTS & JUMPS

Sprint events like the 100- and 200-meter dash require linear acceleration and maximum velocity ability at a high level. To perform these movements and reduce the likelihood of injury, a linear-focused warm-up must be implemented, with an emphasis on lower body flexibility and a strong core.

Recreational Athletes: *Perform one set per session.*   **Elite Athletes:** *Perform two sets per session.*

	PAGE	EXERCISE	DISTANCE/REPS
	p. 48	Toe Walk	10 yards
	p. 49	Heel Walk	10 yards
	p. 50	Side Ankle Walk	10 yards
	p. 89	Ankle Taps	10 yards
	p. 57	Hamstring Handwalk—Inchworm	10 yards
	p. 58	Spiderman Crawl	10 yards
	p. 105	Scorpion	10 yards
	p. 79	Power Skips	30 yards
	p. 77	Repeated Squat Jumps	10 yards
	p. 92	Squat Jump Sprint	30 yards
	p. 84	A-Walk, Skip, Run Progression	40 yards
	p. 86	B-Walk, Skip, Run Progression	40 yards

TRACK AND FIELD—THROWS

Throwing events such as discus, shotput, hammer and javelin are events that require explosive single-repetition activities. This results in a need for explosive power production through dynamic range of motion in multiple planes of motion.

Recreational Athletes: Perform one set per session.   *Elite Athletes: Perform two sets per session.*

	PAGE	EXERCISE	DISTANCE/REPS
	p. 50	Side Ankle Walk	10 yards
	p. 67	Overhead Squat Progression	10 yards
	p. 57	Hamstring Handwalk—Inchworm	10 yards
	p. 58	Spiderman Crawl	10 yards
	p. 105	Scorpion	10 yards
	p. 62	Rotational Walking Lunge	20 yards
	p. 66	Lateral Lunge	20 yards
	pp. 102–104	Hugs/Cheerleaders/Wipers Combo	10 yards
	p. 101	Dynamic Empty Can	10 yards
	p. 76	Countermovement Squat Jumps	20 yards
	p. 56	Upper Body Handwalk	10 yards
	p. 72	Lateral Pass	20 yards

VOLLEYBALL

Volleyball focuses on multi-directional movements and a high percentage of vertical movements. Warm-ups for volleyball need to focus on dynamic range of motion for the lower back, core and legs, with a secondary focus on range of motion at the shoulder.

Recreational Athletes: Perform one set per session.　　　　*Elite Athletes: Perform two sets per session.*

	PAGE	EXERCISE	DISTANCE/REPS
	p. 48	Toe Walk	10 yards
	p. 49	Heel Walk	10 yards
	p. 50	Side Ankle Walk	10 yards
	p. 85	Overhead Squat	10 yards
	p. 57	Hamstring Handwalk—Inchworm	10 yards
	p. 58	Spiderman Crawl	10 yards
	p. 84	A-Walk, Skip, Run Progression	10 yards
	p. 75	Split Jumps/Lunge Jumps*	20 yards
	p. 94	Burpee Sprint	20 yards
	p. 76	Countermovement Squat Jumps	20 yards
	p. 77	Repeated Squat Jump	20 yards
	p. 96	10-Yard Movement Sequence	10 yards

Add Hugs, Wipers and/or Cheerleaders to lunge exercise to warm-up upper body as well.

WRESTLING

Wrestling requires great strength and flexibility in the entire body. This requires an overall warm-up that emphasizes movements and positions that focus on unusual and non-traditional positions.

Recreational Athletes: Perform one set per session.   *Elite Athletes: Perform two sets per session.*

	PAGE	EXERCISE	DISTANCE/REPS
	p. 49	Heel Walk	10 yards
	p. 51	Knee to Chest Walk	10 yards
	p. 57	Hamstring Handwalk—Inchworm	10 yards
	p. 58	Spiderman Crawl	10 yards
	p. 105	Scorpion	10 yards
	p. 62	Rotational Walking Lunge*	20 yards
	p. 68	Sumo Squat Walk	20 yards
	p. 69	Low Squat Walk	20 yards
	p. 95	Lateral Shuffle	20 yards
	p. 94	Burpee Sprint	20 yards
	p. 96	Upper Body Handwalk	20 yards

*Add Hugs, Wipers and/or Cheerleaders to lunge exercise to warm-up upper body as well.

part 3:
the
exercises

toe walk

Objective: Develops strength, functional range of motion and stability around the ankle joint and strengthens the calf muscles.

STARTING POSITION: Stand tall with good posture, keeping your shoulders back.

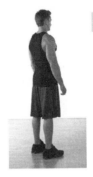

starting position

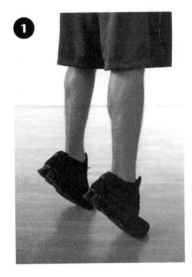

1 Raise both heels and balance on the balls of your feet.

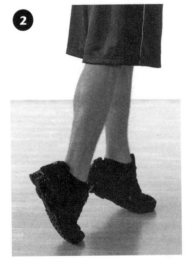

2 Step forward with your left leg and push into the ground with the ball of your left foot, trying to extend up onto your toes. This movement will activate the contraction of the calf muscles.

Step forward with your right leg and repeat the process. Continue alternating legs.

heel walk

Objective: Develops strength, functional range of motion and stability around the ankle joint. Also strengthens the muscles around the shin bone to help reduce the likelihood of shin splints.

STARTING POSITION: Stand tall with good posture, keeping your shoulders back.

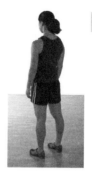

starting position

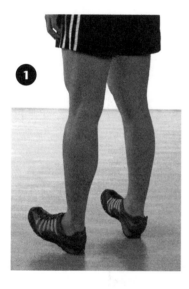

1 Raise your toes off the ground.

2 Step forward with your left leg and push your body-weight into your heel, pointing your toes to the sky. This movement will activate the anterior tibialis (the muscle that runs down the front of your leg from your knee to the ankle area).

Step forward with your right leg and repeat the process. Continue alternating legs.

side ankle walk

Objective: Develops strength, functional range of motion and stability around the ankle joint. Also focuses on the muscles, tendons and ligaments that can help prevent the most common ankle sprains (inversion ankle sprains, wherein the ankle rolls over the outside of the foot).

STARTING POSITION: Stand tall with good posture, keeping your shoulders back.

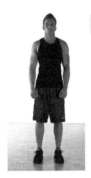

starting position

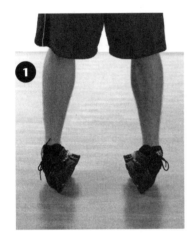

1 Invert your feet so that you're balancing on the outer edges of both feet.

2 Step forward with your right leg and position your body weight on the outside of your right foot, which will result in the arch of your right foot coming of the ground.

Step forward with your left leg and repeat the process. Continue alternating legs.

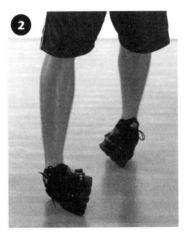

Objective: Develops functional range of motion in the lower back and hip flexor muscles while also improving dynamic balance and postural control.

STARTING POSITION: Stand tall with good posture, keeping your shoulders back.

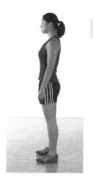

starting position

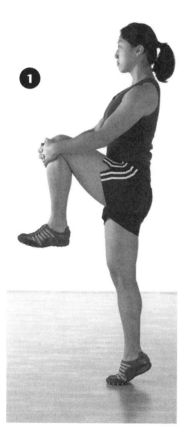

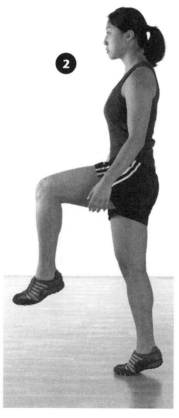

1 Lift your left knee and grab it with both hands, pulling it high and close to your chest. At the same time, rise up high on your right toes, keeping an erect posture from your heel all the way up through the top of your head. Hold this position for approximately two seconds.

2 Slowly release your knee and take a step forward with your left leg to repeat the process.

Continue alternating legs.

walking quad stretch

Objective: Develops flexibility in the hip flexor and quadriceps muscles while also improving single-leg balance.

STARTING POSITION: Stand tall with good posture, keeping your shoulders back.

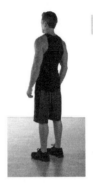

starting position

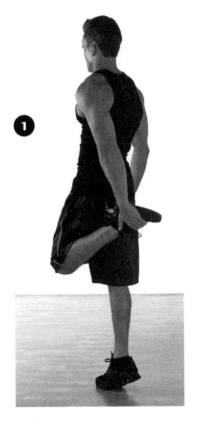

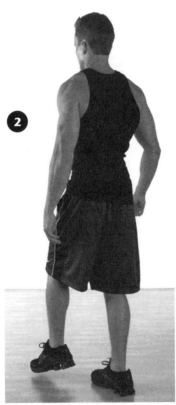

1 Bend your left knee and grab your left foot behind you with your left hand. At the same time, rise up onto the toes on your right foot. Hold this position for approximately two seconds.

2 Release your left foot, let the left leg step forward and repeat the process with your right leg.

Continue alternating legs.

knee to shoulder lateral walk—frogger

Objective: Develops functional range of motion in the hips, specifically the external hip rotators, while developing multi-limb coordination.

STARTING POSITION: Stand tall with good posture, keeping your shoulders back. Extend your arms at shoulder height straight out to the sides, palms facing forward.

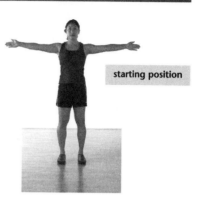

starting position

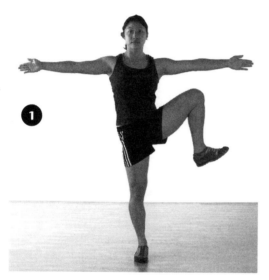

1 Flex your left hip and, as it starts to rise, externally rotate it to bring your knee up toward your armpit.

2 As your left leg comes down, perform the same motion on your right side.

Continue alternating legs.

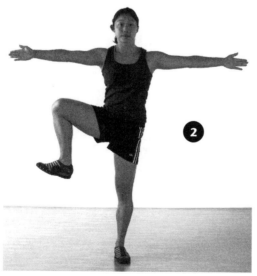

ADVANCED

For more of a challenge, try this with a skipping motion, which will require a greater degree of coordination and also induce a greater plyometric response.

one-leg walking opposite—ostrich

Objective: Develops functional range of motion, balance and multi-limb coordination.

STARTING POSITION: Stand tall with good posture, keeping your shoulders back.

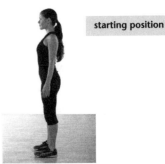

starting position

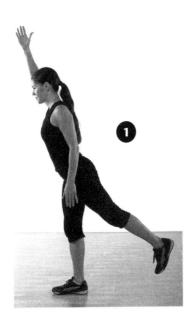

1–2 Step forward with your right leg, maintaining a slight bend in your knee while extending your right arm straight above your head and slowly extending your left leg straight behind you. At the same time, extend your left arm out to the side.

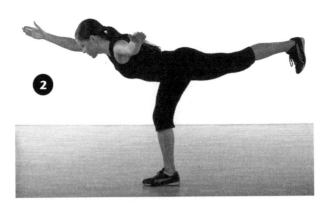

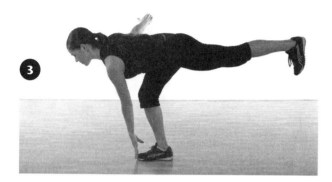

3 Keeping a neutral spine and a forward gaze (as opposed to looking down at the ground), slowly bend at the waist and move your left hand forward to touch your right toe. Hold this position for approximately two seconds. You may extend your right arm to the side for balance. You should feel a stretch through your glute and hamstring muscles.

4 Slowly reverse the movement back to starting position.

Repeat on the other side and continue alternating legs.

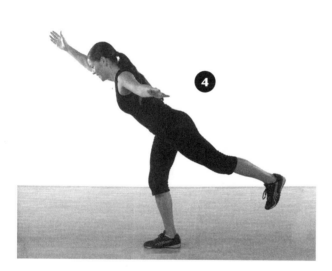

BEGINNER

The "Ostrich" is challenging for most individuals. The "Airplane" is somewhat easier: Instead of touching your right hand to your left toes and vice versa, hold your arms out to the sides in a "T."

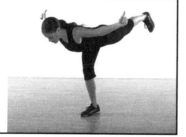

upper body handwalk

Objective: Develops upper body strength and endurance, specifically in the muscles that maintain stability of the shoulder.

STARTING POSITION: Place your hands on the floor and step your feet back so that you're in a high push-up position.

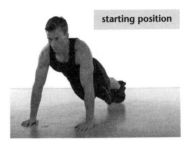
starting position

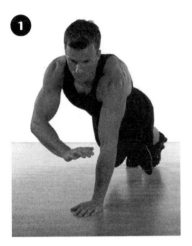
1

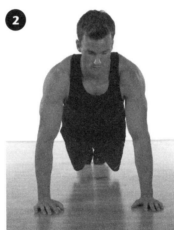
2

1–3 Maintaining a good push-up position, walk your hands to your left. Repeat to your right.

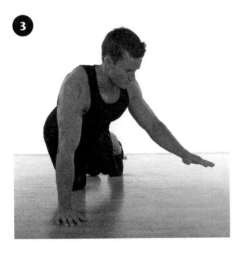
3

hamstring handwalk—inchworm

Objective: Develops functional range of motion in the hamstrings and lower back while increasing strength in the arms, shoulders and core.

STARTING POSITION: Keeping your legs straight, place your hands as far forward on the ground as possible. Make sure your heels stay on the ground and that your arms are extended.

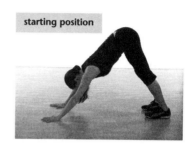

starting position

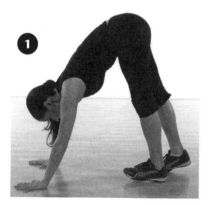

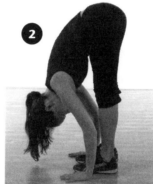

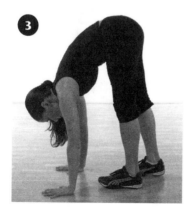

1–2 While keeping your back and legs straight, slowly walk your feet as close as possible to your hands without allowing your knees to bend. You will feel a stretch in your hamstrings and through your lower back.

3 Once you've walked your feet as close as possible to your hands, slowly walk your hands out as far as possible into starting position.

Continue this sequence.

spiderman crawl

Objective: Develops functional range of motion in the hips and lower back while increasing strength in the arms, shoulders and core.

STARTING POSITION: From a standing position, take a small to medium step forward with your left leg at approximately 45 degrees. Bend at your waist and knee to crawl forward, maintaining a neutral spine and walking your hands forward toward your left foot/knee. Keep your eyes looking straight ahead.

starting position

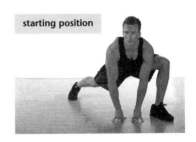

1–3 Slowly walk your hands across to your right as your right leg slowly comes forward.

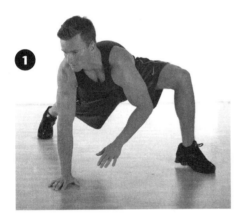

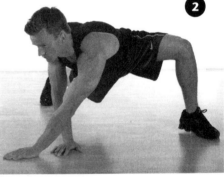

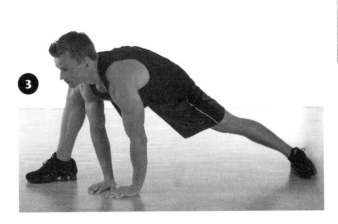

straight-leg march

Objective: Develops hamstring and lower back flexibility

STARTING POSITION: Stand tall with good posture, keeping your shoulders back. Extend your arms out in front of you at shoulder height.

starting position

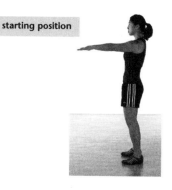

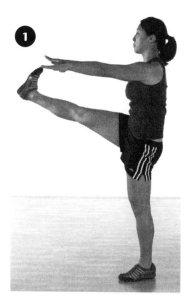

1 Extend your right leg straight out in front of you to touch your fingers. Try not to bend your knee. Focus on maintaining a tall posture, squeezing your bellybutton to your spine and keeping your shoulders back.

2 Lower your right leg to the ground and repeat on the left.

Continue alternating legs.

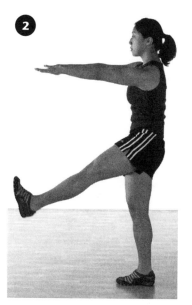

VARIATION

The Straight-Leg Skip is the same general movement pattern but the speed of the movement is increased and instead of a walking movement, this is a skipping exercise. This is an advanced movement and requires a good base level of functional flexibility in the lower back and hamstring muscles.

Objective: Develops functional range of motion in the hip flexors while improving strength in the quadriceps, glutes and core.

STARTING POSITION: Stand tall with good posture, keeping your shoulders back and your hands on your opposing elbows at shoulder height (think *I Dream of Jeannie*).

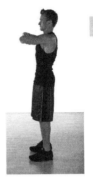
starting position

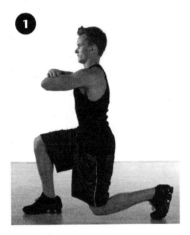

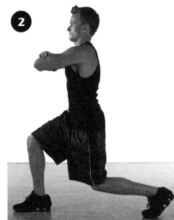

1 Step forward with your right foot and bend your back leg until your knee is about 1 to 3 inches from the ground, directly under your left hip, and your right knee is at a 90-degree angle. Your right knee should be directly above your right ankle.

2 Push off with your left leg to bring it forward into the next lunge.

Continue alternating legs.

VARIATIONS

This lunge can be performed with many different upper body positions, such as with your arms straight above your head and straight out to the side at shoulder height (T position). By altering the arm placement and upper torso position, you can stretch the lower back and core to varying degrees and throughout different planes of motion.

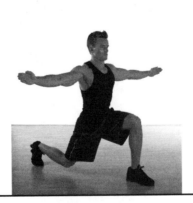

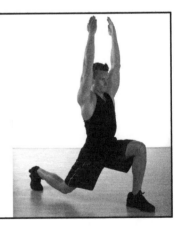

straight-leg walking lunge

Objective: Improves range of motion in the hip flexors while improving strength in the quadriceps, glutes and core.

STARTING POSITION: Stand tall with good posture, keeping your shoulders back and your hands on your opposing elbows at shoulder height (think *I Dream of Jeannie*).

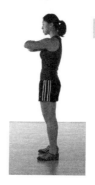

starting position

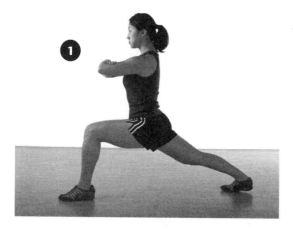

1 Keeping your right leg straight, step your left leg forward and bend your knee until it's at a 90-degree angle. Your left knee should be directly above your left ankle.

2 Push off with your right leg to bring it forward into the next lunge.

Continue alternating legs.

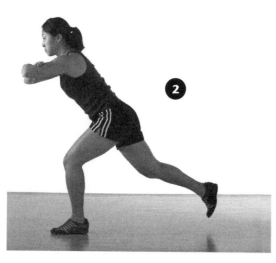

rotational walking lunge

Objective: Develops functional range of motion in the hip flexors and rotational muscles of the core while improving strength in the quadriceps, glutes and core.

STARTING POSITION: Stand tall with good posture, keeping your shoulders back and your hands on your opposing elbows at shoulder height (think *I Dream of Jeannie*).

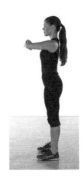

starting position

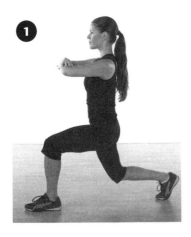

1

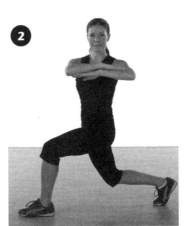

2

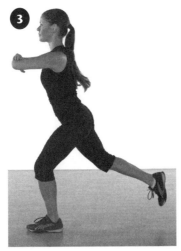

3

1–2 Step forward with your left foot and bend your back leg until your knee is about 1 to 3 inches from the ground, directly under your right hip, and your left knee is at a 90-degree angle. Your left knee should be directly above your left ankle. As you lower your weight, slowly rotate to the left, twisting from your waist over your left leg.

3 Push off with your right leg to bring it forward into the next lunge, this time rotating to the right.

Continue alternating legs.

VARIATIONS

This exercise can be performed with different upper-body arm positions, which will influence muscle recruitment of the core to different degrees.

Clasping your hands straight above your head will elongate the spine and give the lower back muscles (erector spinae and multifidus) a greater stretch.

Reaching your hands straight above your head without clasping you hands will work your obliques and hip rotators to a greater extent.

Reaching the opposite hand (to the front leg during the lunge) straight above your head and rotating will increase the stretch of the muscles of the upper back and mid-back region.

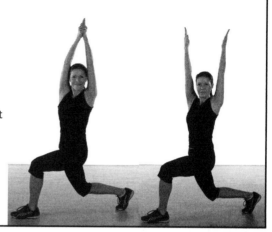

elbow to knee lunge

Objective: Develops functional range of motion in the hip flexors, glutes and external hip rotators.

STARTING POSITION: Stand tall with good posture, keeping your shoulders back and your hands on your opposing elbows at shoulder height (think *I Dream of Jeannie*).

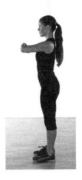

starting position

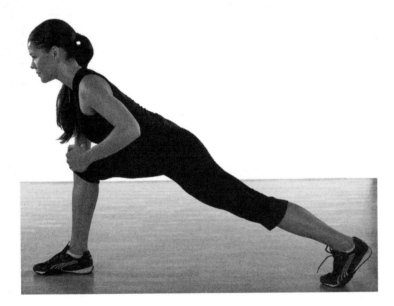

1 Step forward with your right foot, keeping your back leg straight. Your right knee should be bent 90 degrees and be directly above your right ankle. As you lower your weight, keep your back straight and slowly push your right elbow against the inside of your right knee. Hold this position for approximately two seconds.

Push off with your left leg to bring it forward into the next lunge. Continue alternating legs.

VARIATION

This can also be done with a bent back leg. In this case, the back knee should be about 1 to 3 inches from the ground, directly beneath the back hip.

knee-to-chest hold into lunge

Objective: Develops balance, coordination and strength in the core and lower body.

This is a combination of a Knee to Chest Walk and the Linear Walking Lunge.

STARTING POSITION: Stand tall with good posture, keeping your shoulders back.

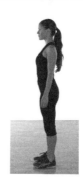

starting position

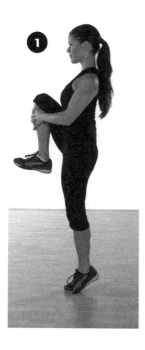

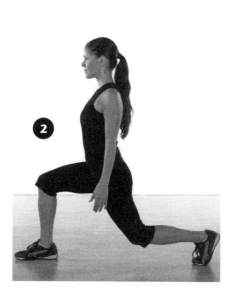

1 Lift your right knee and grab it with both hands, pulling it high and close to your chest. At the same time, rise up high on your left toes, keeping an erect posture from your heel all the way up through the top of your head. Hold this position for approximately two seconds.

2 Step forward with your right foot and bend your back leg until your knee is about 1 to 3 inches from the ground, directly under your left hip, and your right knee is at a 90-degree angle. Your right knee should be directly above your right ankle.

lateral lunge

Objective: Develops hip mobility in a lateral direction while also dynamically stretching the glutes, hamstrings and groin.

STARTING POSITION: Assume an athletic stance.

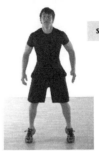

starting position

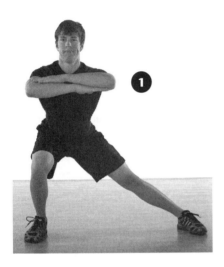

1 Step to the right side with your right leg, keeping your foot facing forward. Slowly lower your weight back into your hips and drop your hips in line (parallel) with your right knee, which is bent approximately 90 degrees. Hold this position for approximately two seconds, making sure that your spine is erect and your shoulders are back with good posture.

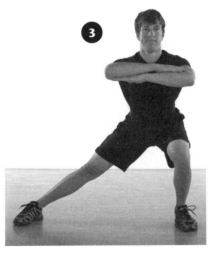

2–3 Bring your left foot in under your center and repeat this movement on the left side.

Perform a number of these on the left side, return to starting position, and then perform the same movement on the right side.

Objective: Increases hamstring range of motion, hip mobility, and scapula strength, flexibility and stability.

STARTING POSITION: Holding a bar, stand with your feet shoulder-width apart. Keeping your legs straight, lower the bar until it is directly over your shoelaces.

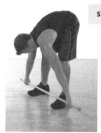
starting position

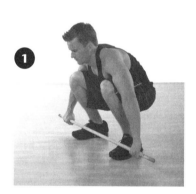
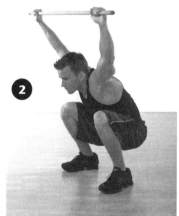

1 Lower into a deep squat.

2–3 Raise the bar overhead, straighten your back, and look forward.

4 Slowly stand upright, keeping your arms extended overhead.

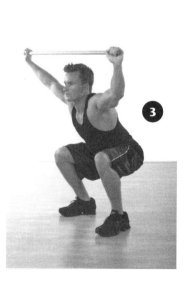
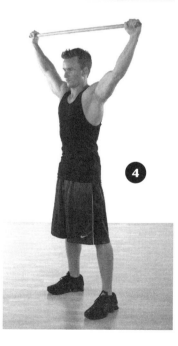

sumo squat walk

Objective: Develops hip mobility while strengthening the glutes, quadriceps and core.

STARTING POSITION: Stand tall with your feet shoulder-width apart, keeping your shoulders back.

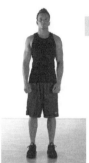

starting position

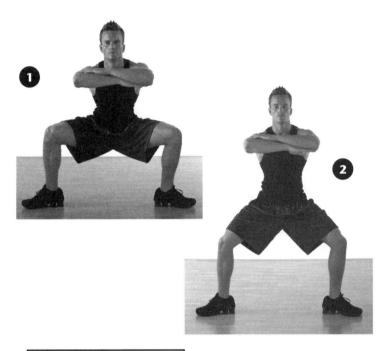

1 Place your hands on your opposing elbows at shoulder height and step to the side with your right leg, pointing your foot away from your body (to the right). As your right foot goes out, turn your left foot to point away from your body (to the left). When both feet are pointing outwards, put all your weight back into your glutes and pretend that you're sitting in a chair while maintaining an erect spine and keeping your shoulders back. Attempt to go as low as possible while maintaining good upper body posture and without "breaking" at the core. Hold this position for approximately two seconds.

2 Stand upright to return to starting position, rotate your body 180 degrees and perform the same movement.

Repeat the process, working on increasing the depth of each sumo squat every time.

ADVANCED

For an extra challenge, raise both arms up to the ceiling as you sink into your squat. This position will raise your center of mass, thereby increasing difficulty.

low squat walk

Objective: Develops strength in the hips, lower body and core.

STARTING POSITION: Lower into a full, deep squat position with your hips at least parallel with the ground and your knees slightly wider than shoulder-width apart. Ideally you should be able to descend lower than knee height while still maintaining a strong, activated core region and erect spine. Place your hands on your opposing elbows at shoulder height (think *I Dream of Jeannie.*)

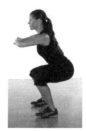

starting position

1 While maintaining the low squat and a low center of gravity, take a small step in front of your body with your right leg.

2 Repeat with your left leg.

Continue alternating legs.

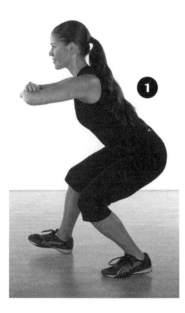

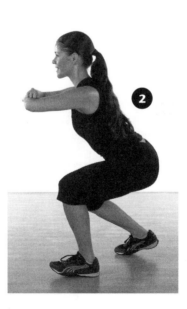

figure-4 squat

Objective: Develops increased range of motion in the external hip rotators while strengthening the glutes and quadriceps. This movement also develops multi-limb coordination and single-leg balance.

STARTING POSITION: Stand tall with your feet shoulder-width apart, keeping your shoulders back. Place your hands on your opposing elbows at shoulder height (think *I Dream of Jeannie.*)

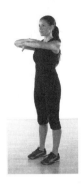

starting position

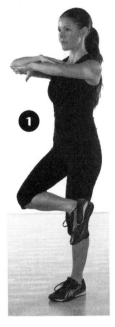

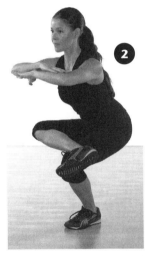

1–2 Lift your right leg, externally rotate your hip and bend your knee so that you can rest the outside of your right ankle on your left thigh. Slowly lower your left hip into a one-leg squat position. This exercises stretches the right external hip rotators and right glute while strengthening the left leg and hip.

3 Return to starting position and rotate your body 180 degrees to perform the movement on the other side.

Repeat the process, working on increasing the depth of each figure-4 squat while maintaining a strong upper body position.

glute ham bridge

Objective: Increases range of motion in lower back, hamstrings and glutes.

STARTING POSITION: Lie on your back with your arms along your sides. Bend your knees and place your feet on the floor close to your buttocks.

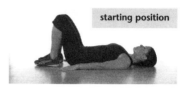

starting position

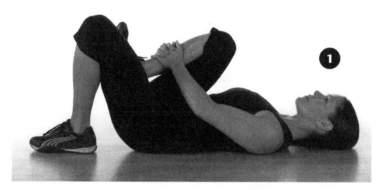

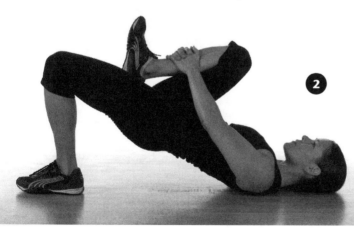

1 Maintaining good posture through your neck and back, hug your right knee to your chest.

2 Press into your left foot and lift your hips until your body makes a nice line from knee to shoulder blades.

Return to starting position and repeat to the other side.

lateral pass

Objective: Increases rotational range of motion in lower back and hips and improves multi-limb coordination.

STARTING POSITION: Assuming an athletic stance, stand back to back with your partner while holding a medicine ball in front of you.

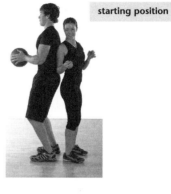

starting position

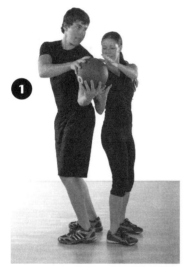

1–2 Keeping your feet in place, twist to your left and pass the ball to your partner.

3 Twist to the other side to receive the ball from your partner.

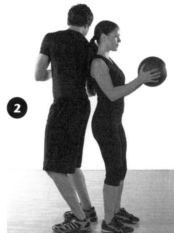

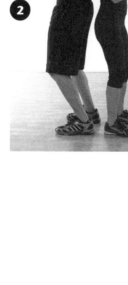

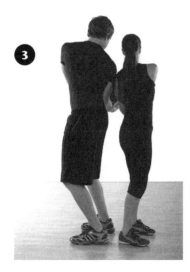

Objective: Improves range of motion of latissimus dorsi and increases upper body strength and flexibility.

STARTING POSITION: Stand back to back with your partner while holding a medicine ball in front of you.

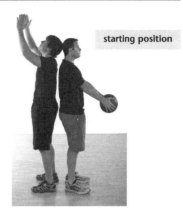

starting position

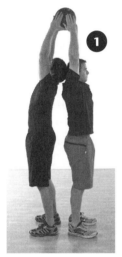

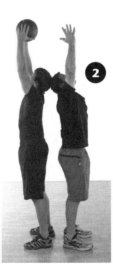

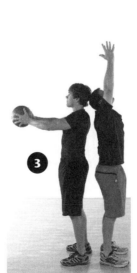

1–2 Reach the ball directly overhead and slightly behind you so that your partner can receive it.

3 Your partner returns the action.

ankle flips

Objective: Develops functional range of motion and explosive power in the muscles around the ankle joint. Also develops force-producing capabilities of the shin (anterior tibialis) and calf muscles (gastroc-soleus complex).

STARTING POSITION: Stand tall with your feet shoulder-width apart, keeping your shoulders back.

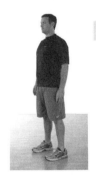

starting position

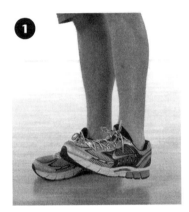

1 Keeping your left leg straight, take one step with your left leg, pointing your left foot to the sky (dorsiflexion).

2 Immediately and forcefully fire the foot down into the ground. As this foot makes ground contact, take a step with your right leg, pointing your foot to the sky.

Continue the cycle while maintaining a strong core and great upper body posture.

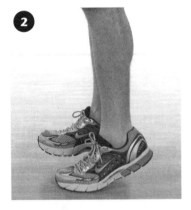

split jumps/lunge jumps

Objective: Develops explosive power throughout the entire lower body while improving single-leg strength, balance and coordination.

STARTING POSITION: Stand tall with your feet shoulder-width apart, keeping your shoulders back.

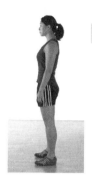

starting position

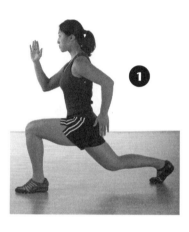

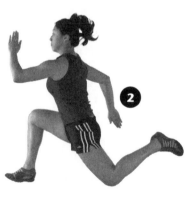

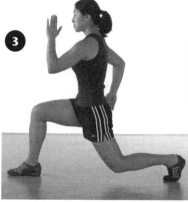

1 Step forward with your left leg into a lunge position, with your front knee bent 90 degrees and in line with your ankle. Bend both arms approximately 90 degrees.

2–3 From this lunge, explode up vertically, thrusting your hips and arms up while keeping a 90-degree angle at your elbows. In the air, your back leg (right) will come forward to become your front leg when landing back into a lunge.

As you land with your right leg in front, immediately explode straight back up as high as possible. Continue alternating legs.

countermovement squat jumps

Objective: Develops explosive power throughout the entire lower body.

STARTING POSITION: Stand tall with your feet shoulder-width apart, keeping your shoulders back.

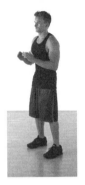

starting position

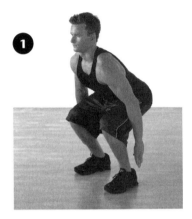

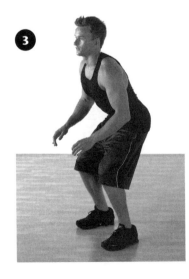

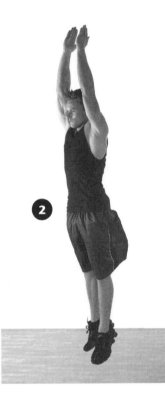

1–2 Squat down until your knees are bent 90 to 135 degrees; without any pause at the bottom of the movement, immediately reverse direction and explode up as high as possible in a straight vertical line, utilizing power transfer from the ground through the ankles, knee and hip joints (known as "triple extension"). Reach your arms high.

3 Gently bend your knees as you land to allow for effective shock absorption; hold the landing for two seconds. This hold at the landing works on your ability to decelerate, which is important in the prevention of injuries during training and helps limit the likelihood of injury during athletic competition.

Return to starting position and repeat the movement.

repeated squat jumps

Objective: Develops explosive power throughout the entire lower body while improving repeatable plyometric ability.

STARTING POSITION: Assume an athletic stance.

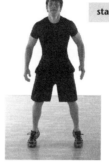

starting position

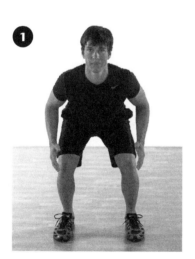

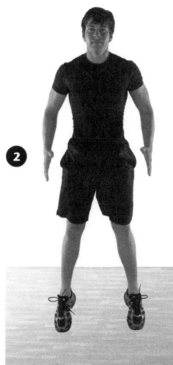

1–2 Squat down until your knees are bent 90 to 135 degrees; without any pause at the bottom of the movement, immediately reverse direction and explode up as high as possible in a straight vertical line, utilizing power transfer from the ground through the ankles, knee and hip joints (known as "triple extension").

As you land, immediately explode straight back up as high possible.

concentric squat jumps

Objective: Develops a combination of concentric strength and power in the lower body.

STARTING POSITION: Stand tall with your feet shoulder-width apart, keeping your shoulders back. Squat down until your knees are approximately 90 degrees and pause for three to five seconds while maintaining an erect spine and strong core position.

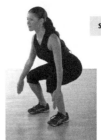

starting position

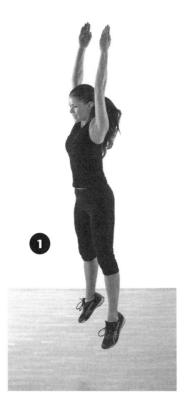

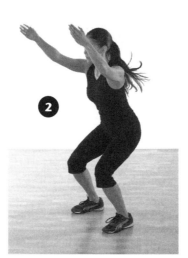

1 Explode up as high as possible in a straight vertical line, utilizing power transfer from the ground through the ankles, knee and hip joints (known as "triple extension"). Reach your arms high.

2 Gently bend your knees as you land to allow for effective shock absorption; hold the landing for two seconds. This hold at the landing works on your ability to decelerate, which is important in the prevention of injuries during training and helps limit the likelihood of injury during athletic competition.

Return to starting position and repeat the sequence.

Objective: Develops a combination of power in the lower body and increased range of motion in the hip flexors and calves.

STARTING POSITION: Stand tall with your feet shoulder-width apart, keeping your shoulders back.

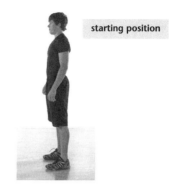
starting position

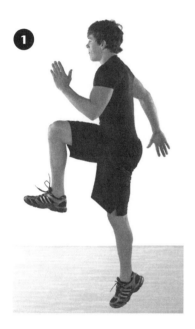
1

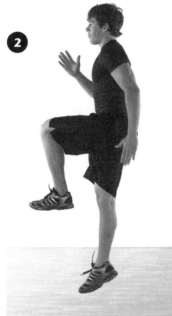
2

1 Leading with your right leg, skip as high as possible by pushing your right knee up towards your right hip, simultaneously bending your left arm 90 degrees. Your left leg should remain straight and your right elbow should be slightly bent by your side.

2 Land on the ball of your left foot and repeat the skipping motion with your opposite arm and leg. This is considered one repetition.

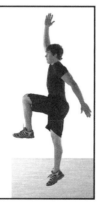

VARIATION
For increased upper body involvement, try extending one arm up to the ceiling as you skip.

high-knee run

Objective: Develops increased range of motion in the hip flexors, lower back and calves, while developing dynamic balance and stability in the core and hips.

STARTING POSITION: Stand tall with good posture, keeping your shoulders back.

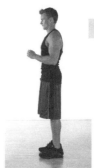

starting position

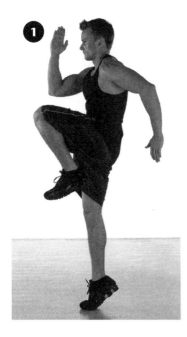

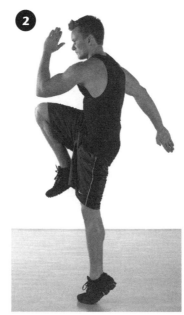

1 Start the run by raising your right leg, bending your knee slightly and pulling your toe to the sky (dorsiflexion). Allow the thumb of your left hand (keeping an approximate elbow angle of 90 degrees in your arm) to track from your hip to your nose. Increase the degree of hip flexion while maintaining an erect upper-body position and strong core.

2 Repeat on the other side.

Continue the cyclical motion of the running movement, focusing on very short ground contacts with the ball of the foot.

jump jump sprint

Objective: Develops explosive lower-body power and reduces ground reaction time.

STARTING POSITION: Assume an athletic stance.

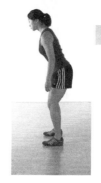

starting position

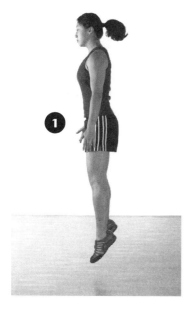

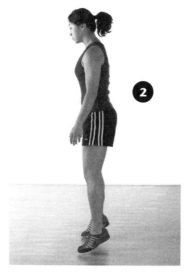

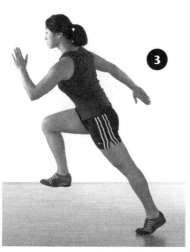

1–2 Take two small broad jumps forward.

3 As you land after the second jump, immediately explode into a sprint, focusing on an efficient acceleration position. In an efficient acceleration position, your body should lean approximately 45 degrees forward, as measured from the heel of the back leg up through the spine; your front knee is up in front of your body with your toes pointing to the sky. Sprint for 10 meters.

Walk back to the starting position.

Repeat the sequence. For endurance, allow 30 seconds of recovery. For speed, strength and power, allow two to three minutes of recovery.

backpedal

Objective: Improves dynamic balance and range of motion of the hips and lower back while concurrently strengthening the quadriceps and hamstrings in a backward direction.

STARTING POSITION: Assume an athletic stance.

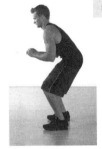

starting position

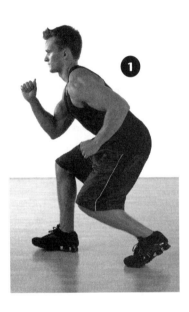

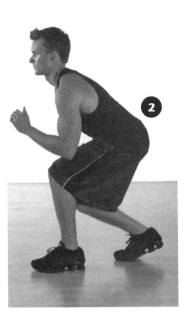

1–2 Leading with your hips and bringing your knees up, move rapidly backward by pushing your legs back down toward the ground. Arm movement should be similar to that used when running in the forward direction, while maintaining a low center of gravity and a stable upper body position.

backward run

Objective: Develops increased range of motion in hip extensors, hip flexors and lower back muscles. This movement also helps to balance the development of opposing muscles to a regular linear-running movement gait.

STARTING POSITION: Assume an athletic stance.

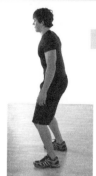

starting position

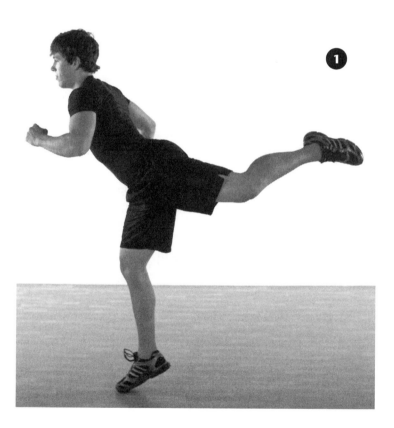

1 Keeping your core tight and upper body erect, run backward by leading with your feet. Push your heels backward away from your body, trying to cover as much distance as possible per step.

a-walk, skip, run progression

Objective: Develops linear-acceleration sprinting mechanics through the training of hip flexion, body forward propulsion and effective stride length.

STARTING POSITION: Stand tall with your feet shoulder-width apart, keeping your shoulders back.

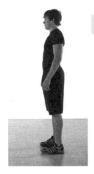

starting position

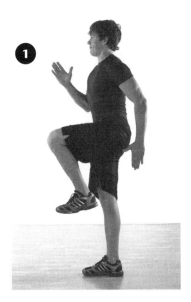

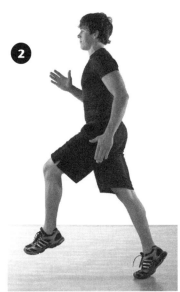

1 Step forward with your left leg, allowing your right elbow to bend approximately 90 degrees and your left arm to move backward. Emphasize a knee-up and toe-up position in preparation for an aggressive and forceful pushing of the left foot into the ground underneath the hip. Pointing the toe up maintains a positive shin angle to help with the forward hip position.

2 Forcefully drive the left leg down into the ground, utilizing efficient hip extension.

VARIATION

Once the mechanics are learned effectively, gradually increase the tempo to a skipping movement; for the more advanced speed athlete, this movement can be increased a running tempo. *Caution:* One common error that occurs once athletes progress from the walk to the skip is losing control of proper core and hip position.

overhead squat

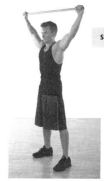

starting position

Objective: Develops core and lower-body strength as well as functional range of motion at the shoulder and upper extremities.

STARTING POSITION: Stand with your feet just wider than shoulder-width apart. Hold a broomstick or weighted bar at arm's length overhead.

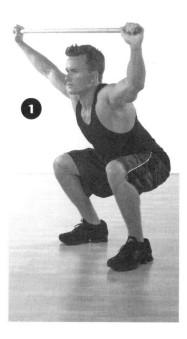

1 Keeping your elbows straight, inhale slowly and bend your knees and lower your hips with a slight backward/down path, with the goal of reaching at or below knee level. Hold the position at the bottom of the movement for a few seconds, focusing on a strong core and an upright body position.

2 From the bottom position, exhale and slowly stand upright while maintaining a strong core.

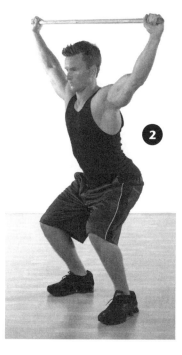

b-walk, skip, run progression

Objective: Develops ground recovery mechanics during sprinting. This is a major performance objective for athletes during high- or maximum-velocity movements.

STARTING POSITION: Stand tall with your feet shoulder-width apart, keeping your shoulders back.

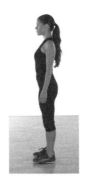

starting position

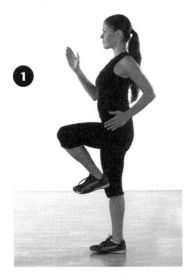

1 Lean forward and bend your left knee to lift your heel upward and slightly in front of your body to a height equal or greater than your right knee.

2–3 Immediately accelerate your left thigh downward while straightening your leg and pulling your thigh backward under the left hip in a clawing motion. During this movement, keep your foot dorsiflexed (toe pointed to the sky).

Continue alternating legs.

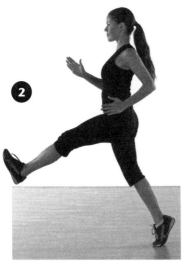

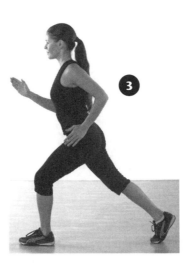

Objective: Develops plyometric ability in the lower body and improved stretch-shortening capabilities while increasing the ability to generate, as well as absorb, high forces.

Caution: This movement produces high forces at the ankle, knee, hip and lower back of the landing leg during each ground contact. This is an advanced movement for athletes who've had appropriate training before attempting the movement.

STARTING POSITION: Stand tall with good posture, keeping your shoulders back.

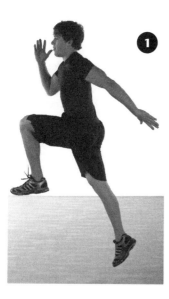

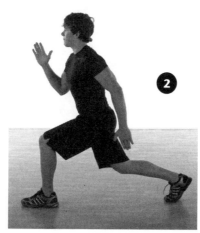

starting position

1 Raise your left leg, bend your knee slightly and pull your toe to the sky (dorsiflexion). Bend your right elbow 90 degrees and allow your thumb to track from your hip to your nose. Increase the degree of hip flexion while maintaining an erect upper body position and strong core. As your left leg comes off the ground, a forward propulsion brings your right leg off the ground; maintain a straight-leg position from the hip to the ankle at an approximate 45-degree angle from the ground. The goal of each bound is to gain great distance.

2 Land on your left foot, utilizing a bent-leg position to provide shock absorption upon landing. Your goal is to limit ground contact time before the next cyclical movement. Focus on very short ground contacts with the ball of your foot.

straight-leg bound

Objective: Develops plyometric ability in the lower body, specifically in the area around the ankles.

Caution: This movement produces high forces at the ankle, knee, hip and lower back of the landing leg during each ground contact. This is an advanced movement for athletes who have had appropriate training and have progressed appropriately.

STARTING POSITION: Stand tall with good posture, keeping your shoulders back.

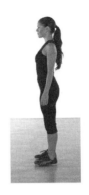

starting position

1 Raise and extend your left leg in front of your body, keeping your core strong and shoulders retracted while maintaining an erect upper body position. Allow your body to lean back slightly and your right arm to bend 90 degrees.

2 When your hip is extended between 30 and 50 degrees, forcefully push the ball of your left foot back into the ground via contraction of the hip extensors.

Alternate legs.

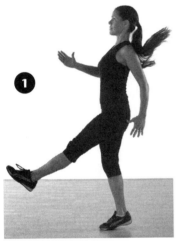

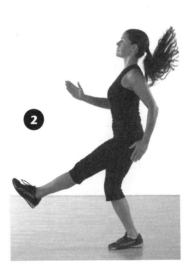

Objective: Develops power production at the foot and smaller muscles that aid in explosive ground contact.

STARTING POSITION: Stand tall with good posture, keeping your shoulders back.

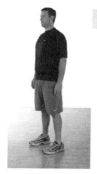

starting position

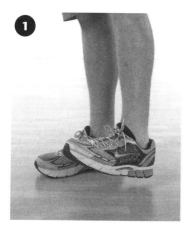

1 While maintaining an erect body position from your heels through your head, pull the toe of your left foot to the sky (via ankle dorsiflexion) and lift your heel off the ground via slight hip flexion; do not bend your knee.

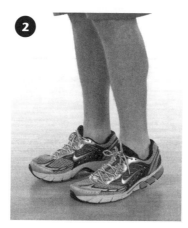

2 Explosively push your foot down into the ground by contracting your gastroc-soleus complex (plantarflexion).

Repeat with your right leg, alternating ground contact over a 5- to 10-yard distance, focusing on explosive force into the ground and limiting the time that each foot is in contact with the ground.

quick feet sprint

Objective: Develops short, quick, explosive ground contacts followed by an immediate response to a stimulus, working on "first-step" quickness and initial acceleration.

You'll need a coach or training partner for this drill.

STARTING POSITION: Assume an athletic position with weight evenly distributed between left and right legs.

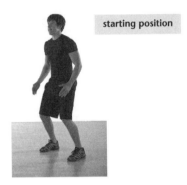

starting position

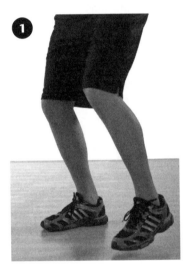

①

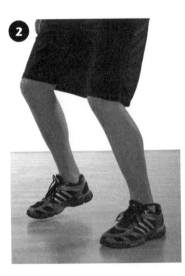

②

1–2 Alternate touching your left and right feet to the ground at rapid pace (the "quick feet drill").

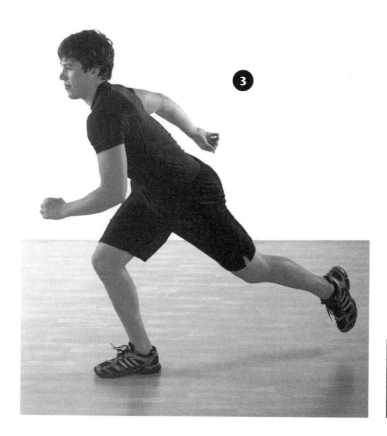

3 When your coach or training partner presents a visual or auditory stimulus, explode from the quick feet drill into a linear sprint focused on acceleration technique and large force generation into the ground on each step forward. Also attempt to limit your time spent on the ground (this increases power production).

VARIATION
The Quick Feet Sprint can also be performed with lateral movements.

squat jump sprint

Objective: Develops triple flexion followed by triple extension at the ankle, knee and hip joints, followed by an explosive ground reaction response into an acceleration position. (In an efficient acceleration position, your body should lean approximately 45 degrees forward, as measured from the heel of the back leg up through the spine; your front knee is up in front of your body with your toes pointing to the sky.)

STARTING POSITION: Assume an athletic position with weight evenly distributed between left and right legs.

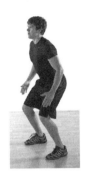

starting position

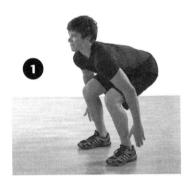

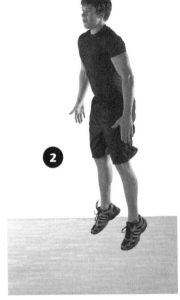

1–2 Perform a squat jump by bending at the hips; when your hips are in line with your knees (parallel to the ground), explode up.

3 At the top of the jump, focus on decelerating the landing. As you land, immediately drive your leg forward into an acceleration position and sprint forward for 10 yards.

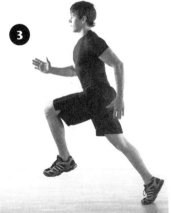
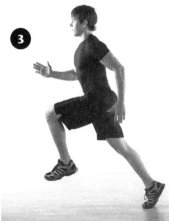

VARIATION

To increase the height of the jump, you can also drive your arms up as high as possible and extend your hips, knees and ankles (triple extension).

Objective: Develops repeatable explosive power and plyometric ability followed by explosive acceleration.

STARTING POSITION: Assume an athletic position with weight evenly distributed between left and right legs.

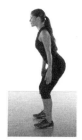

starting position

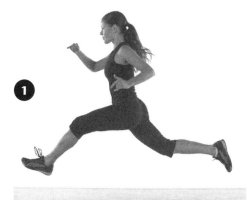

1

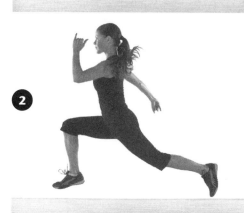

1–3 Perform three single-leg jumps (alternating legs) forward, focusing on both height and depth during each jump.

4 After the third jump, landing on the opposite foot that you started jumping with, push forward into an acceleration position and sprint 10 yards.

2

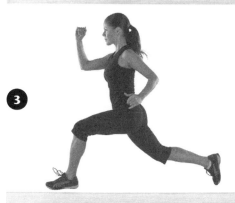

3

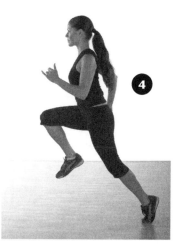

4

burpee sprint

Objective: Develops lower body power, plyometric ability and explosive acceleration.

STARTING POSITION: Place your hands on the floor and step your feet back so that you're in a high push-up position.

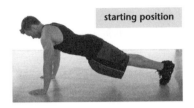
starting position

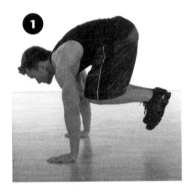

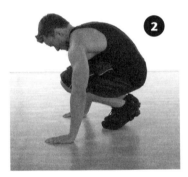

1–3 Push your hands into the ground and explosively bring your knees to your chest to explode upward into an acceleration sprinting position and drive forward, accelerating for 10 yards.

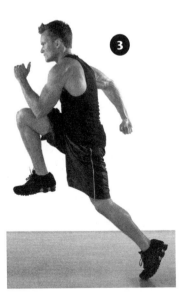

lateral shuffle

Objective: Develops strength and stability in the muscles that initiate and control lateral movement.

STARTING POSITION: Assume an athletic stance.

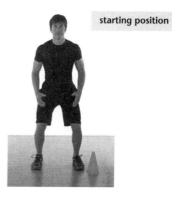

starting position

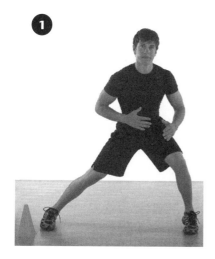

1

1 Keeping your hips low and facing forward the entire time, shuffle to your left for 10 meters. While shuffling, always keep your feet shoulder-width apart while also maintaining a low center of gravity.

2 Shuffle to your right.

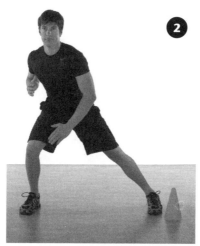

2

10-yard movement sequence

Objective: Warms up the body for linear and lateral movements.

Perform each of the following movements at about 80 percent of maximum speed for 10 yards. Do one, turn and then perform the next movement in the sequence.

STARTING POSITION: Assume an athletic position.

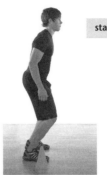

starting position

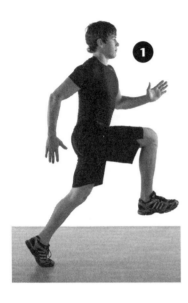

1 Perform a linear run.

2 Perform a Lateral Shuffle (see page 95) toward your right side.

3 Perform a Lateral Shuffle toward your left side.

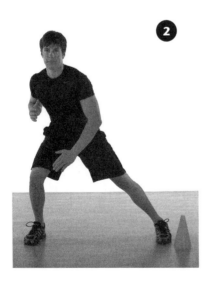

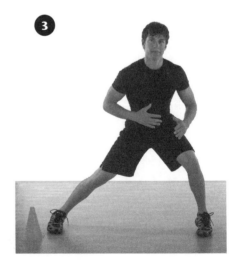

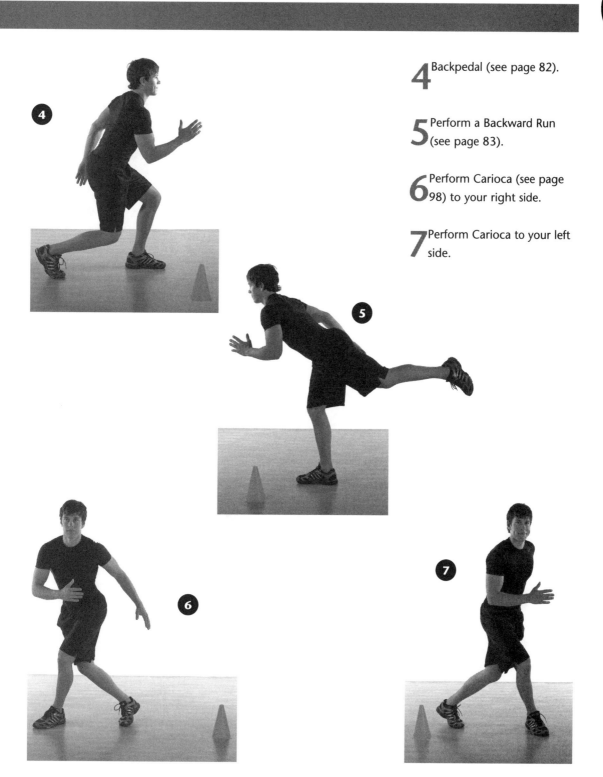

4 Backpedal (see page 82).

5 Perform a Backward Run (see page 83).

6 Perform Carioca (see page 98) to your right side.

7 Perform Carioca to your left side.

carioca

Objective: Increases dynamic range of motion of the hip rotators, while also stretching the groin, hamstrings and core muscles.

STARTING POSITION: Assume an athletic position and extend both arms out to the sides at shoulder height.

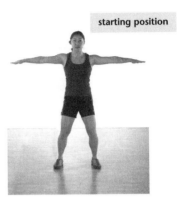

starting position

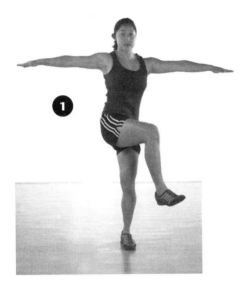

1–2 Step your right leg in front of and across (laterally) your left leg.

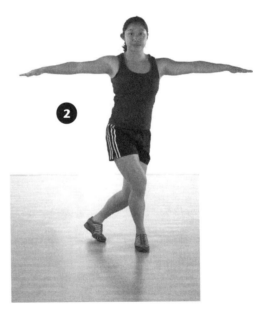

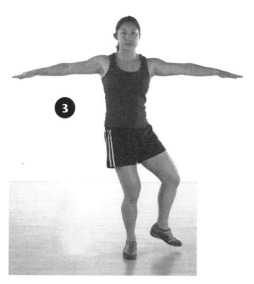

3 Moving in the same lateral direction, step your left leg to the left to return to starting position.

4 Step your right foot in back of and across your left leg. Continue this progression of stepping behind to stepping in front in one lateral direction and then repeat in the other direction back to your starting location.

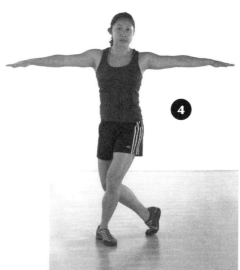

HIGH-KNEE VARIATION

This uses a similar movement pattern but exaggerates the cross-over step and increases the height of the knees above the waist.

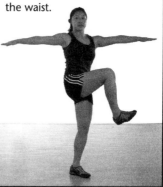

high-knee lateral skip

Objective: Improves hip, knee and ankle mobility and improves lateral movement patterns.

STARTING POSITION: Assume an athletic stance and extend both arms out to the sides at shoulder height.

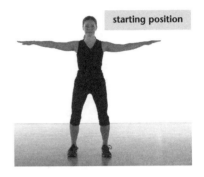
starting position

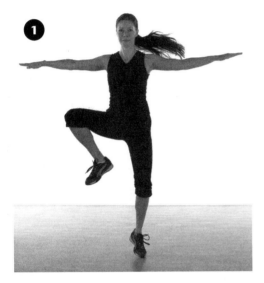

1 With the intention of moving to the right, explosively bring your right knee to your armpit and then explosively return your right leg to the ground, making contact with the ball of the foot.

2 As your right foot touches the ground, perform the movement with your left leg.

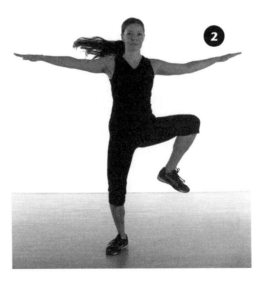

dynamic empty can

Objective: Improves shoulder strength and endurance, specifically the suprasptinatus muscle of the rotator cuff.

STARTING POSITION: Stand tall with good posture, keeping your shoulders back and your arms along your sides. Internally rotate both arms so that the backs of your hands turn in towards your thighs.

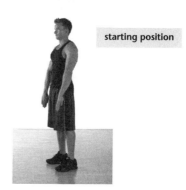

starting position

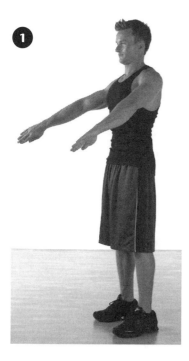

1

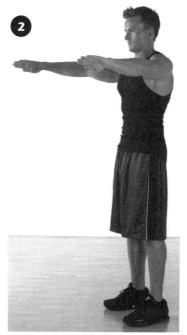

2

1–2 Raise your arms approximately 60 degrees, to just below shoulder height, continuing to internally rotate your arms as if to empty a can.

Repeat using a controlled tempo.

VARIATION

This exercise can also be performed with a light weight (typically 1 to 3 pounds).

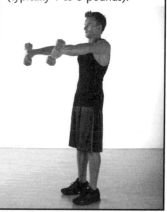

hugs

Objective: Improves dynamic range of motion of the shoulders and chest.

STARTING POSITION: Stand tall with good posture, keeping your shoulders back, and extend your arms in front of you at shoulder height.

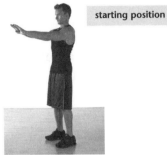

starting position

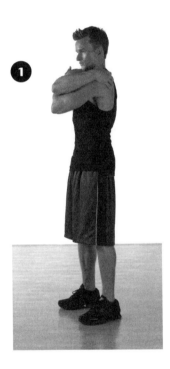

1 Wrap your arms around your body and try to grasp the back of your opposing shoulder.

2 Reverse the movement by taking your arms back and squeezing your shoulder blades together.

Repeat using a controlled tempo.

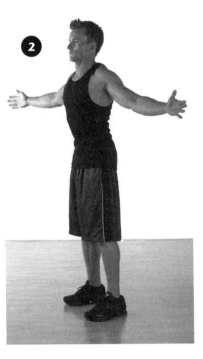

VARIATIONS

This exercise can be performed concurrently with many lower-body movements such as lunges, skips and ankle walks to speed up the warm-up or to challenge the athlete from a balance and coordination perspective.

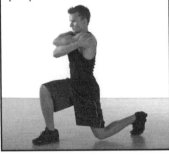

Objective: Improves dynamic range of motion of the shoulders and chest.

STARTING POSITION: Stand tall with good posture, keeping your shoulders back.

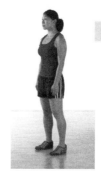

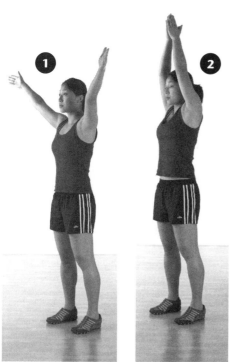

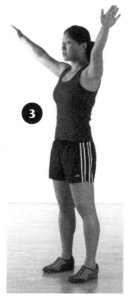

1–2 Slowly raise both arms out to your sides and straight above your head, touching both palms at the top of the movement.

3–4 Lower your arms out to the sides and then down by your waist in a circular arc.

Repeat the movement at varying speeds.

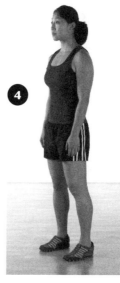

VARIATIONS

This exercise can be performed concurrently with many lower body movements such as lunges, skips and ankle walks to speed up the warm-up or to challenge the athlete from a balance and coordination perspective.

wipers

Objective: Improves dynamic range of motion of the shoulders.

STARTING POSITION: Stand tall with good posture, keeping your shoulders back. Extend your arms straight out in front of your body.

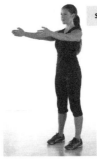

starting position

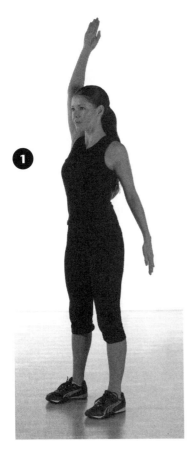

1

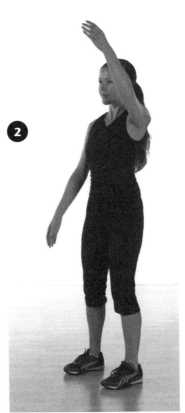

2

1 Slowly raise your right arm while simultaneously lowering your left arm.

2 Change direction and repeat.

VARIATIONS

This exercise can be performed concurrently with many lower-body movements such as lunges, skips and ankle walks to speed up the warm-up or to challenge the athlete from a balance and coordination perspective.

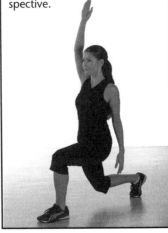

scorpion

Objective: Increases range of motion in the lower back muscles while also increasing the stability of the entire core.

STARTING POSITION: Lie face-down on the floor with your legs long and your arms extended straight out to the sides.

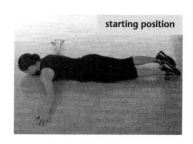

starting position

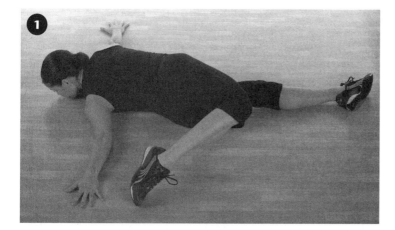

1 Slowly take your right leg across your body to the left and hold for 10 seconds. The goal is to place your right toes as close to your left hand as possible.

2 Repeat to the other side.

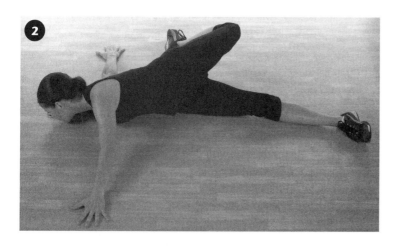

endnotes

1. Shellock, F.G., and W.E. Prentice. "Warming up and stretching for improved physical performance and prevention of sports related injuries." *Sport Medicine* 1985; 2:267-268.

2. Smith, C.A. "The warm-up procedure: To stretch or not to stretch. A brief review." *Journal of Orthopaedic & Sports Physical Therapy* 1994; 19:12-17.

3. DeVries, H.A. "The 'looseness' factor in speed and O^2 consumption of an anaerobic 100-yard dash." *Research Quarterly* 1963; 34(3):305-313.

4. Kokkonen, J., A.G. Nelson, and A. Cornwell. "Acute muscle stretching inhibits maximal strength performance." *Research Quarterly for Exercise & Sport* 1998; 69:411-415.

5. Nelson, A.G., I.K. Guillory, A. Cornwell, and J. Kokkonen. "Inhibition of maximal voluntary isokinetic torque production following stretching is velocity specific." *Journal of Strength & Conditioning Research* 2001; 15(2):241-246.

6. Nelson, A.G., and J. Kokkonen. "Acute ballistic muscle stretching inhibits maximal strength performance." *Research Quarterly for Exercise & Sport* 2001; 72(4):415-419.

7. Avela, J., H. Kyröläinen, and P.V. Komi. "Altered reflex sensitivity after repeated and prolonged passive muscle stretching." *Journal of Applied Physiology* 1999; 86(4):1283-1291.

8. Fletcher, I.M., and B. Jones. "The effect of different warm-up stretch protocols on 20-m sprint performance in trained rugby union players." *Journal of Strength & Conditioning Research* 2004; 18(4):885-888.

9. Fowles, J.R., D.G. Sale, and J.D. MacDougall. "Reduced strength after passive stretch of the human plantar flexors." *Journal of Applied Physiology* 2000; 89(3):1179-1188.

10. Nelson, A.G., N.M. Driscoll, M.A. Young, and I.C. Schexnayder. "Acute effects of passive muscle stretching on sprint performance." *Journal of Sports Sciences* 2005; 23(5):449-454.

11. Young, W., and S. Elliott. "Acute effects of static stretching, proprioceptive neuromuscular facilitation stretching, and maximum voluntary contractions on explosive force production and jumping performance." *Research Quarterly for Exercise & Sport* 2001; 72(3):273-279.

12. Young, W.B., and D.G. Behm. "Effects of running, static stretching and practice jumps on explosive force production and jumping performance." *Journal of Sports Medicine and Physical Fitness* 2003; 43:21-27.

13. Cornwell, A., A.G. Nelson, and B. Sidaway. "Acute effects of stretching on the neuromechanical properties of the triceps surae muscle complex." *European Journal of Applied Physiology* 2002; 86:428-434.

14. Cornwell, A., A.G. Nelson, G.D. Heise, and B. Sidaway. "The acute effects of passive muscle stretching on vertical jump performance." *Journal of Human Movement Studies* 2001; 40:307-324.

15. Wilson, G.J., A.J. Murphy, and J.F. Pryor. "Musculotendinous stiffness: Its relationship to eccentric, isometric, and concentric performance." *Journal of Applied Physiology* 1994; 76(6):2714-2719.

16. Evetovich, T.K., N.J. Nauman, D.S. Conley, and J.B. Todd. "Effect of static stretching of the bicep brachii on torque, electromyography, and mechanomyography during concentric isokinetic muscle action." *Journal of Strength and Conditioning Research* 2003; 17(3):484-488.

17. Knudson, D.V., G.J. Noffal, R.E. Bahamonde, J.A. Bauer, and J.R. Blackwell. "Stretching has no effect on tennis serve performance." *Journal of Strength and Conditioning Research* 2004; 18(3):654-656.

18. Garrett, W.E. "Muscle flexibility and function under stretch." In *Sports and Exercise in Midlife*,

eds. S.L. Gordon, X. Gonzalez-Mestre, and W.E. Garrett. Rosemont, IL: American Academy of Orthopaedic Surgeons, 1993:105-116.

19. Hunter, D.G., and J. Spriggs. "Investigation into the relationship between the passive flexibility and active stiffness of the ankle plantar-flexor muscles." *Clinical Biomechanics* 2000; 15(8):600-606.

20. Pope, R.P., R.D. Herbert, J.D. Kirwan, and B.J. Graham. "A randomized trial of pre-exercise stretching for prevention of lower-limb injury." *Medicine & Science in Sports & Exercise* 2000; 32(2):271-277.

21. Comeau, M.J. "Stretch or no stretch? Cons." *Strength and Conditioning Journal* 2002; 24(1): 20-21.

22. Herbert, R.D., and M. Gabriel. "Effects of stretching before and after exercising on muscle soreness and risk of injury: Systematic review." *British Medical Journal* 2002; 325(7362):468-470.

23. Pope, R.P., R.D. Herbert, and J.D. Kirwan. "Effects of flexibility and stretching on injury risk in army recruits." *Australian Journal of Physiotherapy* 1998; 44:165-172.

24. Shrier, I. "Stretching before exercise does not reduce the risk of local muscle injury: A critical review of the clinical and basic science literature." *Clinical Journal of Sport Medicine* 1999; 9:221-227.

25. Shrier, I. "Does stretching improve performance?: A systematic and critical review of the literature." *Clinical Journal of Sport Medicine* 2004; 14(5):267-273.

26. Levine, U., J. Lombardo, J. McNeeley, and T. Anderson. "An analysis of individual stretching programs of intercollegiate athletes." *Physician and Sportsmedicine* 1987; 15:130-136.

27. Shrier, I. "Flexibility versus stretching." *British Journal of Sports Medicine* 2001; 35(5):364.

28. Shrier, I., and K. Gossal. "Myths and truths of stretching." *Physician and Sportsmedicine* 2000; 28(8):57-63.

29. Yeung, E.W., and S.S. Yeung. "A systematic review of interventions to prevent lower limb soft tissue running injuries." *British Journal of Sports Medicine* 2001; 35(6):383-389.

30. Andersen, J.C. "Stretching before and after exercise: Effect on muscle soreness and injury risk." *Journal of Athletic Training* 2005; 40(3):218-220.

31. van Mechelen, W., H. Hlobil, H.C.C. Kemper, W.J. Voorn, and R. de Jongh. "Prevention of running injuries by warm-up, cool-down, and stretching exercises." *American Journal of Sports Medicine* 1993; 21(5):711-719.

32. Macera, C.A., R.P. Pate, K.E. Powell, K.L. Jackson, J.S. Kendrick, and T.E. Craven. "Predicting lower-extremity injuries among habitual runners." *Archives of Internal Medicine* 1989; 149(11):2565-2568.

33. Thacker, S.B., J. Gilchrist, and D.F. Stroup. "The impact of stretching on sports injury risk: A systematic review of the literature." *Medicine & Science in Sports & Exercise* 2004; 36:371-378.

34. Knudson, D. "Stretching during warm-up: Do we have enough evidence?" *Journal of Physical Education, Recreation and Dance* 1999; 70(7):24-27.

35. Kovacs, M.S. "The argument against static stretching before sport and physical activity." *Athletic Therapy Today* 2006; 11(3):24-25.

36. Cornelius, W.L., R.W. Hagemann, and A.W. Jackson. "A study on placement of stretching within a workout." *Journal of Sports Medicine and Physical Fitness* 1988; 28:234-236.

37. Kovacs, M., W.B. Chandler, and T.J. Chandler. *Tennis Training: Enhancing On-Court Performance.* Vista, CA: Racquet Tech Publishing, 2007.

38. Kovacs, M.S. "Is static stretching for tennis beneficial? A brief review." *Medicine and Science in Tennis* 2006; 11(2):14-16.

39. Bergh, U., and B. Ekblom. "Physical performance and peak aerobic power at different body temperatures." *Journal of Applied Physiology* 1979; 46:885-889.

40. Blomstrand, E.V., B. Bergh, B. Essen-Gustavsson, and B. Ekblom. "The influence of muscle temperature on muscle metabolism and during intense dynamic exercise." *Acta Physiologica Scandinavica* 1984; 120:229-236.

recommended reading

Alter, M. *Science of Flexibility* (3rd edition). Champaign, IL: Human Kinetics, 2004.

Andersen, J.C. "Stretching before and after exercise: Effect on muscle soreness and injury risk." *Journal of Athletic Training* 2005; 40(3):218-220.

Chandler, T.J., and L.E. Brown. *Conditioning for Strength and Human Performance*. Baltimore, MD: Lippincott, Williams and Wilkins, 2008.

Kokkonen, J., and J.M. McAlexander. *Stretching Anatomy*. Champaign, IL: Human Kinetics, 2006.

Kovacs, M.S. "The argument against static stretching before sport and physical activity." *Athletic Therapy Today* 2006; 11(3):24-25.

Kovacs, M., W.B. Chandler, and T.J. Chandler. *Tennis Training: Enhancing On-Court Performance*. Vista, CA: Racquet Tech Publishing, 2007.

Pope, R.P., R.D. Herbert, J.D. Kirwan, and B.J. Graham. "A randomized trial of pre-exercise stretching for prevention of lower-limb injury." *Medicine and Science in Sports and Exercise* 2000; 32(2):271-277.

Shrier, I. "Does stretching improve performance? A systematic and critical review of the literature." *Clinical Journal of Sport Medicine* 2004; 14(5):267-273.

Shrier, I. "Stretching before exercise does not reduce the risk of local muscle injury: A critical review of the clinical and basic science literature." *Clinical Journal of Sport Medicine* 1999; 9:221-227.

index

other ulysses press books

Complete Krav Maga: The Ultimate Guide to Over 230 Self-Defense and Combative Techniques
Darren Levine & John Whitman, $21.95
Developed for the Israel military forces, Krav Maga is an easy-to-learn yet highly effective art of self-defense. Clearly written and extensively illustrated, *Complete Krav Maga* details every aspect of the system, including hand-to-hand combat moves and weapons defense techniques.

Ellie Herman's Pilates Workbook on the Ball: Illustrated Step-by-Step Guide
Ellie Herman, $14.95
Combines the powerful slimming and shaping effects of Pilates with the low-impact, high-intensity workout of the ball.

Functional Training for Athletes at All Levels: Workouts for Agility, Speed and Power
James C. Radcliffe, $15.95
Teaches all athletes the functional training exercises that will produce the best results in their sport by mimicking the actual movements they utilize in that sport. With these unique programs, athletes can simultaneously improve posture, balance, stability and mobility.

Plyometrics for Athletes at All Levels: A Training Guide for Explosive Speed and Power
Neal Pire, $15.95
Provides the nonprofessional with an easy-to-understand explanation of why plyometrics works, the sports-training research behind it, and how to integrate plyometrics into an overall fitness program.

Total Heart Rate Training: Customize and Maximize Your Workout Using a Heart Rate Monitor
Joe Friel, $15.95
Shows anyone participating in aerobic sports, from novice to expert, how to increase the effectiveness of his or her workout by utilizing a heart rate monitor.

To order these books call 800-377-2542 or 510-601-8301, fax 510-601-8307, e-mail ulysses@ ulyssespress.com, or write to Ulysses Press, P.O. Box 3440, Berkeley, CA 94703. All retail orders are shipped free of charge. California residents must include sales tax. Allow two to three weeks for delivery.

acknowledgments

In each person's life there are scores of people who have made a profound impact on the direction of one's life. Rarely do we have a forum to say thank you! Fortunately, I have this opportunity to thank my family, mentors and students: my family for their love, support and willingness to allow me to travel along my own path—for that I am grateful; the many mentors who have made impressions that at the time may have been small, but have shaped thoughts, feelings and actions until this day; to my athletes/students and clients— thank you for unknowingly providing the purpose to strive for knowledge, understanding and the desire to improve every day.

about the author

Mark Kovacs is a leading author, presenter, researcher and trainer in the area of human performance enhancement. He was a top-ranked international junior tennis player as well as an All-American and NCAA doubles champion at Auburn University. After playing professionally, he pursued graduate work in tennis-specific research, and earned a graduate degree in exercise science from Auburn University and a Ph.D. in exercise physiology from the University of Alabama. Mark is a certified strength and conditioning specialist through the National Strength and Conditioning Association, a certified health/fitness instructor through the American College of Sports Medicine, a U.S. Track and Field Level II sprints coach, and a USPTA-certified tennis coach. He has personally trained professional athletes in many sports and high school and collegiate stars, as well as individuals from all walks of life. His holistic approach of combining many scientific disciplines into practical, results-driven programs are at the core of each client's individual success. Mark has published and presented more than 50 research papers and abstracts in numerous top scientific journals and at national and international conferences. He is also the co-author of *Tennis Training: Enhancing On-Court Performance* and is an associate editor of the *Strength and Conditioning Journal*. He oversees the strength and conditioning and sport science areas for the United States Tennis Association (USTA). Prior to joining the USTA, Mark was an assistant professor of exercise science and wellness at Jacksonville State University.